Health Care Reform

A Catholic View

For Kathy Cummings

Philip S. Keane, S.S.

Phil Keane
11/4/93

PAULIST PRESS
New York, N.Y./Mahwah, N.J.

Library of Congress Cataloging-in-Publication Data

Keane, Philip S.
    Health care reform : a Catholic view / Philip S. Keane.
        p.   cm.
    Includes bibliographical references and index.
    ISBN 0-8091-3385-7
    1. Medical policy—United States. 2. Medicine—United States—
Religious aspects—Catholic Church.   I. Title.
    RA395.A3K4   1993
    362.1'0973—dc20   93-10275
                                                            CIP

Published by Paulist Press
997 Macarthur Boulevard
Mahwah, New Jersey 07430

Printed and bound in the
United States of America

CONTENTS

Acknowledgments vii
Introduction 1

PART ONE
THE STATE OF U.S. HEALTH CARE TODAY:
PROBLEMS AND PROSPECTS

1. Difficulties with U.S. Health Care Delivery Today 9
2. Other Options and Other Countries 32

PART TWO
THEOLOGICAL AND MORAL REFLECTIONS ON
HEALTH CARE JUSTICE

3. The Human Person as Mortal and Finite 61
4. The Specific Ethics of Care for the Dying 80
5. Building Community:
   Theological and Philosophical Roots 103
6. The Ethics of the Just Community and the Reform of
   Health Care 122

PART THREE
HEALTH CARE REFORM TO COME:
THE SHAPE OF THE FUTURE

7. Theology and the Churches:
   Their Place in the Health Care Debate 153
8. What Should a Reformed Health Care
   System Look Like? 173

Contents

Postscript 195
Endnotes 199
Abbreviations 223
Index 224

To
My Mother and Father

Harriet Sullivan Keane
and
Gerard Francis Keane

ACKNOWLEDGMENTS

This book was written during my 1991–92 sabbatical from St. Mary's Seminary and University. I wish to express my gratitude to both the Society of St. Sulpice and to St. Mary's Seminary for providing me with the opportunity for the sabbatical. In particular, I wish to thank Father Gerald Brown, S.S., Provincial Superior of the American Province of the Society of St. Sulpice, and Father Robert Leavitt, S.S., President-Rector of St. Mary's. Important help in arranging and implementing the sabbatical was also furnished by Anthony Lobo, S.S., Melvin Blanchette, S.S., Louis Reitz, S.S., Rev. Roger McGrath, Susan A. Lemmon, and Theresa McFadden.

I am grateful to Father Thomas Golueke and to the priests and staff of St. Pius X parish in Baltimore for providing me with the comfortable and welcoming space in which I lived for the year. Similarly, the community of the Immaculate Heart Center in Montecito, California made me feel most welcome in the weeks which I spent there.

Sylvia DeVillers, Ann Neale, Thomas F. Schindler, S.S., Patricia Schoelles, S.S.J., and Thomas R. Ulshafer, S.S. all read the manuscript and made very helpful suggestions. I thank them and also acknowledge that I am the one responsible for any shortcomings in the text. David Siemsen and Kathleen Tallent of the Knott Library at St. Mary's Seminary provided valuable assistance in locating needed resources. As with my earlier books, I was much encouraged by the gracious interest of the Paulist Press, especially by Kevin Lynch, C.S.P., and Richard Sparks, C.S.P.

I have been privileged to have many contacts with health care professionals from whom I have learned much about the issues which this book addresses. I would especially like to thank the administrators, employees, and medical staffs of Mercy Medical Center, Baltimore, and Holy Cross Hospital of Silver Spring where I have been honored to serve as a consulting moral theologian for many years.

By coincidence, I completed the text and wrote these acknowledgments on the date of my twenty-fifth anniversary of ordination to the priesthood. Since the priesthood has been such a joy for me, I would also like to thank all those who helped me move to the priesthood and who have been part of my ministry over the years. This is especially true for my mother and father to whom this book is dedicated.

Baltimore, Maryland
May 20, 1992

INTRODUCTION

Recently, Dr. George Lundberg, the editor of the *Journal of the American Medical Association*, wrote that the movement toward health care reform in the United States has now acquired "an aura of inevitability."[1] Some take this notion of inevitability as meaning that we can expect major health care reforms within a year or two. Other more cautious authors argue that, even if health care reform is inevitable, we are still five to seven years away from the full accomplishment of true systemic changes in the way health care is delivered in the United States.[2] However, no serious thinker questions Dr. Lundberg's basic assertion that the United States is headed toward a period of extensive health care reform. A recent public opinion poll has shown that only about ten percent of U.S. citizens think that our health care system is either just fine as it stands or only in need of minor changes.[3]

If we grant that health care reform in the United States is inevitable, there are still enormous questions as to exactly how health care reform ought to be shaped. Speaking as a moral theologian, I would find it most regrettable if health care reform were based solely on economics and pragmatic political considerations. Health care can often touch us at the very core of who we are as human persons. A whole host of questions about human dignity and human rights are part and parcel of the delivery of health care. Thus, it seems essential that health care reform be based on more than economics and politics, even though it is clear that economics and politics should play a crucially important role in the development of policies for health care reform.

This book will be written as an exercise in theological reflection on health care reform. It will explore the major moral and religious issues which can serve as foundation stones for the reform of health care. In its reflections, the book will draw primarily upon the theological/moral tradition of Roman Catholicism. But insights and emphases from other segments of the Christian tradition and from other religious and moral traditions will often be included.

1

The book will be divided into three major sections, with the second section being the lengthiest and most important. The first section will be descriptive in nature and will consist of two chapters. Chapter 1 will describe the major problems which currently beset the health care delivery system in the United States, beginning with the basic fact that on any given day about thirty-seven million Americans have no health insurance. Most of us are aware of at least some of the problems in health care delivery because of our own experiences or because of the experiences of family members and friends. Still, it is appropriate to begin with a focused understanding of the current problems in health care delivery so that we can reflect meaningfully on possible approaches to change.

Chapter 2 will describe some of the important approaches to health care delivery which are found in other countries such as Canada and Great Britain. It will also describe the main features of the dozen or so serious proposals for reform which have so far been introduced in the United States. The purpose of this chapter will be similar to the purpose of the first chapter. Just as we need to know what our current health care system is like before we can reflect theologically, so too we need to have some sense of the realistic possibilities for change so that we can attempt a theological/moral assessment of where we might move in the area of health care reform.

The purpose of the second and longest section of the book will be to articulate the major theological and moral issues which can serve as underpinnings for today's debate about the reform of health care. The second section will be divided into four chapters addressing the different theological issues which are at stake in health care. In Chapter 3, the book will address the meaning of life, the meaning of sickness and suffering, and the meaning of death, all from the viewpoint of our Christian faith in the resurrection of Jesus. Unless we can come to grips with these very basic questions, it seems that we will continue to lack focus in terms of what we are really trying to accomplish through the delivery of health care. In particular, without an adequate sense of the place of death in human life, we humans will struggle to know what health care is all about. Our status as finite creatures with limited resources and a fragile environment will be important in this context, as will our call to be prayerful worshipers of our God.

Chapter 4 will consider the traditional and contemporary ethics of care for the dying. Over the past four centuries, Roman Catholicism has developed a very sound and thoughtful ethic on care for the dying, an ethic which historically has been rooted in the distinction between ordinary and extraordinary means of caring for our life and health. In recent decades there have been some important efforts to articulate the ordinary/extraordinary distinction in more precise terms,[4] and others besides Roman Catholics have joined the debate about the ethics of care for the dying. But Catholicism's basic insight remains in place: we are not obligated to do everything which we might be able to do to prolong biological life. As we shall see, this insight has a very high potential for helping to shape the search for a more just system of delivering health care.

Chapter 5 will be a reflection on who we are as a community of persons who are bonded to one another both naturally and religiously. Who are we to one another? What sorts of loyalties do we owe to one another? What sort of resources does our faith offer us for the building of community? What does our natural humanity require of us in terms of providing for the health care needs of all people? What kind of virtue should we practice in the area of health care? This part of the book will draw heavily on biblical themes such as covenant and love of neighbor.

Chapter 6 will be an effort to specify the nature of human community in terms of traditional moral categories such as human rights, the common good, and distributive justice. These categories are important in themselves and also important in terms of what they tell us about different economic systems such as capitalism and socialism. In its history, Roman Catholic moral theology has developed a disciplined analysis of human community through the use of such categories as distributive justice and human rights. The social encyclicals of the past one hundred years have contributed notably to the development of concepts of justice, the common good, and human rights. Key contributions have also been made by classic thinkers such as Thomas Aquinas and more recent scholars such as John A. Ryan and John Courtney Murray. A review of the Catholic analyses of human rights, justice, and the common good will put us in a much better position to determine whether and how we can make the claim that a reasonable level of health care is a human right.

In addition to looking at justice and rights issues for the community as a whole, this chapter will need to reflect on the role and claims of special groups such as children, elderly persons, the physically handicapped and the mentally retarded. In recent times the Catholic bishops of the United States have placed substantial emphasis on the theme of the "preferential option for the poor."[5] In the context of health care reform, various segments of the human community may be among the poor, even if not all these members are poor in a material sense.

As this brief outline of the second section has shown, Chapters 3 and 5 are more explicitly theological. They address basic questions about human persons in relationship to God: the question about the meaning of life and death, and the question about the nature of human community. Chapters 4 and 6 are more explicitly moral or ethical. Each of these chapters discusses the moral standards or principles which have emerged from the theological insights of the chapters which precede them. The moral principles about care for the dying flow from the theological vision of life and death, and the principles of justice and human rights flow from the theological vision of the nature of human community. In my view, an adequate theological/ moral statement of the foundations for health care reform needs to touch both on matters of fundamental theological vision, and on the question of disciplined ethical standards. In an earlier book I argued that moral theology needs to engage both the left and the right hemispheres of our brains.[6] My hope is that the links between the four theological/moral chapters will help accomplish this.

The third major section of the book will be divided into two chapters. Chapter 7 will analyze the role which religion and morality ought to play in shaping a future health care delivery system. Clearly there are limits to the role of religion. Health care reform involves much more than religious or moral insights. But just as clearly, religious and moral perspectives can contribute much to the debate about health care reform. Questions about religious liberty and about the role of religion in a democratic society will be an important part of this chapter. Only with an adequate sense of what religious/moral insights can and cannot offer could a theologian begin to make any specific suggestions about the shape of health care reform.

Chapter 8 will be something of an exercise in prophecy, and it will be more tentative and probing than the rest of the book. The main question for this chapter will be as follows: In view of our theological/ moral analysis, what would a reformed system of U.S. health care look like? Of the various proposed options for health care reform, which options and which aspects of which options would seem to be most coherent with the moral values which are at stake? There is no simple answer, but hopefully the book can shed some light on the character of a future and more just health care delivery system. The theological and moral reflections of the middle part of the book cannot be left at the level of abstraction. With due hesitancy, practical conclusions about health care reform will be made in the final chapter.

As the outline of the book has shown, my goal is to present an overview of all of the major points at which Catholic theology and health care reform intersect. As an overview, this book will not be a complete investigation of the issues which it treats. The several major themes which I discuss could easily be subject matters for full-length books. This is true of the description of the state of health care today, of the history of Catholic theology and health care, of the church's official moral teachings on health issues, and of the proposals for health care reform. By writing an overview my hope is to show how all the major pieces of the health care reform puzzle fit together for a Catholic theologian. I believe that such an overview is itself a worthwhile project. My hope is that the overview approach will help the informed Catholic, the theology student, the health care professional who is not an ethicist, and the political leader to see how Catholic thought ties in with the debate about health care reform. But I want to acknowledge that, because of my strategy of presenting an overview, there will remain an obvious need for further analysis of many of the specific issues which I treat.

Some of you may be wondering how I as a theologian came to be concerned about health care reform. In my many years of service as an ethical consultant to a number of different hospitals, I have become convinced that in the final analysis the clinical ethical questions (about how to care for a specific dying patient, etc.) are actually relatively easy to resolve. This is especially true if one is working out of the Roman Catholic tradition with its four centuries of reflection on the clinical cases. In speaking of the *relative* ease of addressing the clinical cases, I am not denying that there can be some agonizingly difficult choices on matters such as supplying artificial nutrition/hydration to certain classes of dying patients and on matters such as the course of treatment to be followed in the care of critically ill newborn children. But in these cases at least the framework and principles for decision making are quite clear.

In contrast, my experience has shown me that the reform of our health care delivery system is the single most difficult question which we face today in the field of health care. And, unlike the situation in clinical cases, we seem to be lacking in an adequate framework out of which to address health care reform as a social moral issue. As a Roman Catholic theologian, I believe that the Roman Catholic tradition can help establish such a framework. In particular, I am convinced that the Catholic tradition of distributive justice can have much to offer to our troubled health care delivery system. This tradition teaches that society is responsible for providing each citizen with a basic level of fundamental human goods. Even though this tradition on distributive justice will not be described in detail until later in the book, it will be the foundation for the way in which I discuss every issue, beginning with the descriptive material of the first two chapters. If this book, with its focus on distributive justice and other key theological issues, can help shape the debate about health care reform, and if it can offer some tentative suggestions for actual change, I believe I will have accomplished my purpose.

PART ONE

THE STATE OF U.S. HEALTH CARE TODAY: PROBLEMS AND PROSPECTS

Chapter 1

DIFFICULTIES WITH U.S. HEALTH CARE DELIVERY TODAY

Before we turn to an analysis of the troubles of the U.S. health care delivery system, we need to be clear that the picture of health care delivery in the United States is by no means entirely bleak or negative. If we consider the twentieth century as a whole, or even the second half of the century, it must be acknowledged that health care has made enormous progress. Since 1900 life expectancy has increased by about three decades. The death rate has declined correspondingly. Modes of treatment which were simply undreamed of (such as laser surgery for eye cataracts) have become commonplace. Cures for some diseases (like many forms of tuberculosis) and vaccines for others (like polio) have been discovered. Heart surgery is now routine and, while more remains to be done, there has been substantial progress in dealing with cancer. Many other examples could also be cited. As this chapter unfolds, its focus will be on the problems of health care delivery. But our emphasis on the problems should not cause us to forget medicine's successes. We shall also discover a certain irony in that the successes have sometimes been at least partly the cause of the problems.

With these accomplishments in mind, we turn to the task of a critical commentary on the U.S. health care delivery system. For our purposes, the difficulties which beset the U.S. health care system can be divided into four categories: lack of access to health care, the high cost of health care, stresses and inefficiencies within the health care system itself, and pressures of health care on the U.S. economy as a whole, so that there is a growing negative public assessment of the U.S. health care system. Many sub-issues fall within each of these four categories, and some of the same sub-issues occur in several of the main categories.

LACK OF ACCESS

The Uninsured and Underinsured: Who Are They?

Here we need to start by talking about numbers, about the kind of numbers which our minds can hardly imagine. Most statistical analyses place the number of persons in the United States who have no health insurance somewhere in the mid-thirty million range, with thirty-seven million being a very commonly cited figure.[1] But even this figure, huge though it is, does not tell us the whole story of lack of access to health care. The figure of thirty-seven million is an estimate of those in the United States who lack health care coverage on any given day. Because of job changes, temporary unemployment, etc., many more Americans are without health care insurance at least part of the time. The U.S. Bureau of the Census estimates that in 1986–1988, more than sixty-three million Americans were lacking in health care insurance for at least one month.[2] In addition, the statistics show that the number of uninsured Americans has increased notably during the past decade, from about twenty-six million at the beginning of the 1980s to the present figure of thirty-seven million. The fear of course is that the number of uninsured will continue to increase unless we move to systemic change in the delivery of health care.

Besides those who have no health care insurance, another sizable group of Americans is underinsured. These persons have some coverage, but their coverage is not adequate to meet their health care needs. It is harder to make an accurate assessment of the number of underinsured, but published estimates have placed the figure between fifteen and thirty million. The temporarily uninsured and the underinsured may often be the same persons as they move from one category to the other and back again, a factor which makes it hard to come up with a total number of uninsured and underinsured. However if we make an estimate that on any given day about sixty-five million Americans are either uninsured or underinsured, the conclusion is that about a quarter of the two hundred and fifty million people counted in the 1990 U.S. Census are either uninsured or underinsured.[3] If we subtract those Americans over 65 (who are almost all considered to be insured because of Medicare), the number of uninsured and underinsured under 65 may be more like one-third of the under 65 population. In human terms, this means that practically all of us will have family members or friends who are lacking adequate health insurance. From a theological viewpoint, it seems impossible to accept the number of uninsured and underinsured as being in accord with the demands of distributive justice.

This problem becomes even more explicit when we begin to analyze the uninsured and underinsured by categories such as age, race, economic status and employment, level of education, sex, geographic location, etc. As to age, those least likely to have health insurance are the 19–24 year olds (20% lack coverage all the time with another 18% lacking it part of the time). This creates a concern that these young people may develop health problems which appear minor at present, but which may cause them serious health difficulties later in life.

After the 19–24 year olds, the second most likely group to lack insurance are children, with about 17% lacking coverage. In terms of infants, the United States continues to have a rather high infant mortality rate when compared with a number of other developed countries in the world. It is true that the U.S. infant mortality rate has dropped significantly since 1950. But the rate of decrease in infant mortality has slowed during the past ten years or so, and some of our large cities have actually seen small increases in their infant mortality rates during recent years. Coupled with this data is the fact that, even with the application of very effective neonatal intensive care to some infants, the U.S. ranks only about twentieth among the world's countries in terms of its infant mortality rate.[4] The U.S. also ranks rather poorly on other comparative vital statistics such as the death rate.[5]

About 19% of persons from ages 25–54 lack health insurance, as do 13% of those persons from ages 55–64. This last figure is a matter of concern since persons in this age group are quite likely to begin having more serious health problems than they did earlier in life.[6]

In terms of race, non-Hispanic Caucasians are the least likely to lack health care insurance, but even in this group a disturbingly high 18% are uninsured. About 30% of African-Americans are uninsured, as are 41% of Hispanics.[7] Studies show that African-Americans have a shorter life expectancy, a greater likelihood of having certain major diseases, and a higher infant and child mortality rate (about 1.7 times that of non-Hispanic Caucasian children).[8] Since Hispanics are significantly more likely than African-Americans to be uninsured, the health status of Hispanics is a cause for special alarm, especially since they are the fastest growing segment of the U.S. population. Since a great many Hispanics are rooted in the Roman Catholic tradition, the health of Hispanics should be a matter of special moral and pastoral concern for the Roman Catholic community.

It should come as no surprise that the lack of access to health care and the resulting greater likelihood of health problems are closely linked with both educational and economic status. Those who are poorer and less well educated are much more likely to lack health insurance and to have more serious health problems. Various statistics might be cited in this area, but one key statistic serves to sum things up: only 4.2% of persons with a high family income and a college education consider their health to be only poor or fair, while 46% of persons with a low income and no high school education report their health to be only poor or fair.[9] Later in the book we will have more to say about the relation of the good of health care to other goods such as education, but even the statistics just cited should make us consider the public health benefit of a greater investment in education.

Since persons with low income and little education are significantly more likely than others to be unemployed, the statistics we have just cited also point to the link between unemployment and the lack of health insurance, especially in recessionary times. Shortly we shall see that changing insurance systems have made it increasingly hard for many employed persons to get sufficient health insurance. But the connection between unemployment and lack of access to health care remains an important factor. One of the key reasons many people fear unemployment is that they fear losing their health insurance.

On the subject of gender, men are slightly more likely to be uninsured than women (23% of men vs. 21% of women).[10] One reason for this is that Medicaid provides coverage for many poor women who are pregnant or who have dependent children. In general men find it almost impossible to qualify for Medicaid, while women, partly because they are among our very poor in increasing numbers, are more likely to be able to qualify for Medicaid.

Geographical location also has a significant impact on the access of Americans to adequate health care. In general, doctors seem to concentrate themselves in suburban areas, with the result that both rural Americans and those who live in the center of urban areas can find it difficult to meet their health care needs, even if they are able to pay. Several authors cite the 1980 statistics from Mississippi where fifty-one of the state's eighty-two counties had no obstetrician and fifty counties had no pediatrician.[11] But the problem occurs all over rural America. Advertisements in medical journals very often include pleas from small towns which have put together very attractive packages to recruit physicians. An example of the problem of urban health care availability comes from the city of Chicago which went from having one doctor for every thousand people in 1950 to having one doctor for every four thousand people in 1970.[12] Similar reports can be found for many other urban centers.

Why No Coverage for So Many?
An Assessment of Our Insurance Systems

The last few paragraphs have sketched a profile of just who the uninsured and underinsured Americans are. But now the question is why. Why are there so many uninsured people in our country and why has the number of uninsured increased so significantly in recent years? These questions can be answered, at least in part, by an assessment of the three major sources of health insurance which operate in our country: Medicare, Medicaid, and private health insurance.

MEDICARE

Of the three systems, it seems reasonable to say that Medicare, which provides coverage for older Americans, has been the most effective.[13] Since its passage in the mid-1960s, Medicare has offered at least basic health insurance to all Americans over 65. The hopes of President Truman and others who had earlier pushed for such a system have to some degree been realized. However, even with Medicare, some significant problems need to be noted. Four such problems can be cited here.

First, about a third of the entire annual Medicare expenditure is used to pay for the care of persons who are in their last year of life. Without doubt, much of this expenditure is necessary, but there is also reason to believe that a significant amount of this funding pays for overtreatments, i.e. for technological supports which the Roman Catholic tradition would consider to be extraordinary because they lack the significant benefit which would make them morally obligatory. If such aggressive steps were not covered by Medicare, there would be more resources available to meet the needs of the thirty-seven million uninsured Americans. This issue will be examined more carefully later.

Second, there are gaps in what Medicare provides for our older citizens. Almost everyone who can afford it buys additional insurance to supplement Medicare. The Medicaid system often ends up being used to help the poor elderly pay for long term care, for Medicare's Part B (which covers physicians' services), and for other related health costs, meaning that less Medicaid funding is available for Medicaid's original purposes such as serving poor women and their dependent children.

Third, Medicare has now become politically entrenched to the point that it has become very hard to change it in ways which might make it more socially responsible. In 1988 the U.S. Congress passed and President Reagan signed catastrophic health insurance legislation which imposed an income tax surtax on wealthier Medicare beneficiaries and added $4 to the cost of Medicare Part B for all beneficiaries. The hue and cry from senior citizens' groups was so loud that Congress gave in and repealed the legislation in spite of some of the very important benefits which it provided.

Fourth, Medicare comes across as a bureaucratic jungle for many older Americans. The forms can be difficult to understand. Many people have to deal with two different sets of forms (one for Medicare and one for their private insurance carrier). Older people often deal with several doctors, each of whom may have slightly different practices for dealing with Medicare and with private insurance. Older people worry whether they have been sufficiently reimbursed, and they sometimes even worry that they have been overpaid for a given procedure. Some complexity is inevitable, but surely the system can be made simpler.

MEDICAID

Many people think that Medicaid emerged as something of an afterthought to the Medicare system. If we were going to cover older people, why not cover poor people as well? Over its history, Medicaid has been understood as more of a welfare program than an entitlement program. On the whole, Medicaid has been a less well thought out and less effective program, even though it does provide some significant health care coverage. Three main difficulties can be cited in the current Medicaid system.

First, unlike its approach to Medicare, Congress left much of the decision-making power about Medicaid (such as what level of poverty is required in order to be eligible) in the hands of the states. The result is that, especially in states with weaker tax bases (often southern states and rural states), Medicaid has been much less available than elsewhere. With so many states facing budget crises during the 1991–92 recession, this type of problem is only likely to become worse. Congress occasionally mandates that the states must cover a specific health care need (e.g. the care of poor pregnant women) to a specific level through Medicaid.[14] State officials often find these congressional mandates very difficult since they can threaten Medicaid with bankruptcy and make it all the more difficult for the states to use Medicaid funds to care for the medically indigent.

Second, the funds available to the states for Medicaid are often used for purposes which seem not to have been part of the original intention of the Medicaid legislation. For instance, Medicaid funds are frequently used to provide for long term care for older persons, and to provide coverage for persons with permanent disabilities such as blindness. Surely long term care and care for the disabled are worthy goals. Nonetheless, they are an example of Medicaid's being used to fill the gaps in other programs rather than meeting its basic purpose of providing care for the poor.

The third difficulty with the Medicaid system is that a substantial number of physicians refuse to care for Medicaid patients. This is true for about 20% of all physicians, with the percentages being higher in certain areas of medical specialization. On the other end of the spectrum, there are questions about some of the physicians whose practices involve care for a very high percentage of Medicaid patients. There have been cases of fraud in this area. There seems to be at least some evidence that some physicians with a high Medicaid load are less well educated and less likely to offer the quality of care which non-Medicaid patients have available to them. (Consider for instance the high rate of foreign-educated physicians who are caring for the urban and rural poor.)[15] These points about fraud and competence level are clearly not true of the great majority of those physicians who accept Medicaid patients. But it remains clear that the Medicaid system as a whole has some serious shortcomings.

Later in the book we will take a look at the question of the covenant loyalties which should exist between various human groups including physicians and patients. This theme of covenant loyalty will make us even more concerned about the problem of physicians refusing to care for patients.

PRIVATE INSURANCE

Since Medicare and Medicaid are government programs, many readers might think it only natural that these systems be full of problems. Working from this "government is all messed up anyway" perspective, one might hope that private health care systems would be in considerably better shape. For me, one of the most revealing and disturbing aspects of the research for this book was the discovery of all the difficulties which are currently besetting the private health insurance industry.

The basic problem with private health insurance today can be described as follows. As health care has become more and more expensive, health insurers have taken more and more steps to reduce their expenses by excluding coverage of persons with high-risk health conditions. This means that persons in risky health situations are finding it harder and harder to buy health insurance. Changing jobs, often a humanly desirable step, becomes an action fraught with peril for many persons because of the uncertainty as to whether the new employer's insurance carrier will cover them or refuse coverage because of some pre-existing health condition.[16]

This growing inaccessibility of private health insurance touches all Americans, but it is an especially difficult burden for small businesses which want to provide health insurance for their employees. Small businesses either face very large health insurance premiums, or their small number of employees is seen as such a risky pool that they cannot buy employee insurance at any price. Many small businesses are trying to ameliorate this situation by making lower cost health maintenance organizations (HMOs) or preferred provider organizations (PPOs) available to their employees, with the employees being asked to pay extra if they need a higher level of coverage. But these steps do not really solve the problem, and in the end some small businesses are simply unable to buy any health care insurance. If we accept the old notion that small businesses are the heart of the American economic way of life, the crisis in private health insurance affordability becomes all the more regrettable.

A number of states have sought to address the private health insurance crisis by creating public high risk pools for those persons who cannot qualify for coverage and by taxing the insurance companies to pay for this high risk coverage. While such efforts have been of some help, the number of persons enrolled in such pools is low, and the problem of excluding persons from coverage because of pre-existing health conditions remains very real.

In one sense, it seems only natural that, in an age of ever rising health care costs, insurance companies would seek to cut their expenses by excluding coverage of persons who are likely to be quite expensive to insure. From another viewpoint, however, it can seem a bit incredible that insurers, whose mission is to protect persons from the risk of costly health care problems, would only protect persons whose risk is low. In many of the European countries, for instance, health insurance operates with a strong sense of covenantal responsibility to all people so that exclusions for pre-existing conditions would seem to be unthinkable.[17] In our country, with its climate of frequent corporate takeovers and its emphasis on profit rather than on mission and product quality, the exclusionary practices of insurance companies seem to fit right in with many of our other business practices.

In fairness to U.S. insurance companies, the cost of health care has become enormously high. It may be too much to expect the insurance companies to spread this cost among their customers without our country at the same time taking some meaningful social steps to help manage the cost of health care more effectively.

WHY DOES HEALTH CARE COST SO MUCH?

The first part of this chapter focused on the millions of Americans who have no health care coverage and on the limits of existing public and private insurance mechanisms. A crucial factor in the lack of access we have just reviewed is the high cost of health care. If health care were not so costly, we would have much less trouble in making a reasonable level of access to health care available to all persons. We need therefore to examine some of the root factors which make health care so expensive. In the long run our ability to develop a more just system of health care delivery will depend significantly on our ability to control the costs of health care.

There are many factors which help bring about the high cost of health care in the U.S. Here we will review seven of these factors: medical technologies, specialization, salaries, the fee-for-service system and the psychology of health care insurance, defensive medicine, fear of death and medical utopianism, and our failure to emphasize preventive medicine.

Medical Technologies

The first major reason why health care is so costly is the ever higher cost of medical technologies. Machines like CT scanners, MRIs (magnetic resonance imagers), etc., can cost vast sums of money, both for development and for production. The only items of similar or greater cost for which our society pays are some of the types of hardware used in the aerospace and defense industries. The cost of items such as MRIs also raises questions of efficiency and distribution. In their desire to compete with one another, hospitals may be tempted to acquire more of these technologies than a given geographical area really needs. Government regulations and regional agreements between medical centers help reduce these distributional inefficiencies, but the problem of inefficient distribution remains as part of today's health care scene.

Without doubt, many of these costly medical technologies can accomplish wonderful things in the world of health care. But the ever growing cost of medical technologies may gradually raise a difficult ethical question. Can we as a society truly afford to pay for every medical technology? Or might we have to set some priorities by determining which technologies we most surely need and by deciding, with regret, that we cannot afford to develop some other technologies? The moral implications of these questions will be addressed when we discuss health care rationing in Chapter 6.

Specialization

A second factor in the cost of health care today is the growing profusion of medical specializations both at the level of physicians and at the level of support personnel such as technicians, therapists, etc. Precisely because of all the advances in medicine, more and more personnel are required to make today's medical services available to patients. Typical patients today may have several different physicians involved in their care, along with a wide range of support personnel. In earlier times, so many patients had their health care needs addressed by a much smaller care team, with the focus being on the role of the family doctor. Even with the current revival of interest in family medicine, medical specialization and the increased cost of paying for it are hallmarks of our health care system.

Financial Compensation

A third element contributing to the high cost of health care today is the relatively high level of financial compensation received by many doctors and other high level health care professionals. It is important that this point not be overemphasized, since it contributes less to the cost of health care than some of the other factors we are considering. It is also important to note that not all doctors are making large amounts of money. (Consider for instance some primary care physicians and some of the doctors in family practice in small towns.) Similarly, we should note that becoming a doctor takes a great deal of time, money, and effort and that health care is a very important human service. Thus it seems reasonable that a strong level of financial compensation be available to doctors and to other high level health care professionals.

But these cautions do not remove the necessity of mentioning financial compensation as an element which contributes to the growing cost of health care. Granting the point that a strong level of compensation is due to doctors and other high level health care professionals, it seems reasonable to argue that, at times, the amount of compensation goes beyond what the notion of a strong level of compensation might justly require. It helps in this context to recall that a substantial part of the cost of medical education and medical research is paid for by the public in the first place. We might also question whether some health care professionals such as marketing experts are truly necessary. Finally, it is interesting to compare what we as a society pay health care professionals with what we pay to persons who offer other very important kinds of human service, persons such as teachers who earn much less in the U.S. Other countries pay groups such as teachers better than the U.S. does, meaning that our scale of values about the relative salaries of various professionals is not the only possible scale which might be used.

In these comments I have not touched upon the compensation of persons who work in health care at lower levels (floor nurses, janitors, housekeepers, laundry personnel, and others). There can fairly frequently be problems of underpayment to such personnel, and these problems will not easily go away in an age when health care institutions are feeling so much pressure to keep costs down. It should go without saying that the traditional Catholic teaching about a living wage ought to apply to all lower level health care personnel.

The Fee-for-Service System and the Psychology of Health Insurance

The term "fee-for-service" refers to the practice of charging patients for each individual medical service which they receive. Here our purpose is not to attack the fee-for-service system as such. Rather the purpose is to point out that the fee-for-service system can have a hidden psychological impact which tends to raise the cost of health care. The psychological impact is this: because doctors and some other health care professionals are aware that their income (or their institution's income) is dependent on the collection of individual fees for specific services, there can be a natural, sometimes subconscious, tendency for doctors and others to think that the more fees they are able to collect, the better they are doing. A similar psychology exists in many other segments of our market-based economy: the higher the sales, the better any business is doing. I am not arguing that this psychology dominates the whole of medical practice. Many doctors are very careful not to overprescribe, overtest, etc. Nonetheless it remains true that the incentives of the fee-for-service system are different from the incentives which occur in other health care delivery settings such as HMOs. To the extent that HMOs have been successful in reducing costs, their success is at least partly due to their avoidance of the fee-for-service system.

As a parallel to these comments about health care providers, it should be noted that the health care insurance system can have a similar effect on the consciousness of those who use insurance to purchase their health care. If the insurance is purchased by one's employer, a person can easily think that, since everything is paid for, he or she should have all possible medical care. Even if a person pays for his or her own insurance, after payment there can be the tendency to think that everything should be done since everything has been paid for. In other words, insurance can take away the incentive to think over whether a given treatment modality is really needed and really in the patient's best interest. It is true that the seriousness of many medical interventions may make us ask these questions even if we have insurance, and insurance systems which involve copayments or other similar devices can help us to make treatment decisions carefully. But in the U.S. where the insurance system worked so well for a number of decades, the very success of the insurance system has lulled many persons into a failure to be more cost conscious in the area of health care.

Defensive Medicine

The fifth reason for the high cost of U.S. health care is often described by the phrase "defensive medicine," i.e. medical practices that are undertaken by a doctor or health care center more out of a fear of lawsuit than out of a true sense of the patient's good. There is a need for some caution in describing this category.[18] To begin with, doctors and hospitals have a clear responsibility to provide their patients with appropriate good quality care. Regrettably there are times when health care providers can fail in exercising this responsibility. At times this can even happen with very fine and well qualified health care providers who are acting out of sincere good will. It is surely true that patients have the right to seek financial compensation when they have been injured by improper use of medical technologies. Thus liability insurance is a normal part of the cost of practicing health care, and there are surely members of the legal profession who handle these health care liability issues in a very caring and professional manner.

However, alongside this reasonable place for liability in health care delivery, many health care professionals have developed an unreasonable fear of lawsuits. The result can be the ordering of all sorts of excess and sometimes costly medical tests and procedures, procedures which are not really necessary for the patient's good but which will serve to protect the caregivers from lawsuits. Coupled with this unreasonable fear of lawsuits is the fact that the extra tests, etc., may be a source of further income for the physicians, or for their associates or colleagues. It is to be hoped that future medical practice can develop clearer standards about which medical tests and procedures are truly necessary. With such clear standards, perhaps the era of defensive medicine can retreat a bit.

The high cost of medical liability insurance has something of a "chicken or the egg" relationship to all the other factors which drive up medical costs. On the one hand, medical liability costs are at least partly a derivative of the high general cost of health care. If we can reduce general health care costs, this may help reduce the cost of liability. But at the same time we do live in a society which seems to grow more and more litigation-oriented, more likely to seek suits in all kinds of life areas. If we can develop a sense of community which is a little less litigation-oriented, this too may help reduce the cost of health care. Some states are trying to address this problem by placing limits on medical malpractice awards, but it may be that a deeper conversion of heart and mind will be necessary before we can truly address all the issues related to defensive medicine.

Another note in this context is that health care professionals could learn to do more to police themselves, more to improve the already existing procedures for licensure and credentialing. Doctors in particular have been in a position of great trust and respect in society for the past several generations. This can make it hard for anyone, even peers, to criticize the work of a doctor. (Similar situations can develop with priests and ministers because of their high social position.) If the health care profession can develop more effective ways of criticizing substandard performances by doctors and other health care professionals, some instances of medical malpractice might be prevented in the first place.

The Fear of Death and Medical Utopianism

The sixth point in our survey of the factors which raise the cost of health care has to do with the contemporary attitude toward death and with the utopian hopes which many place in modern medicine. If we study earlier cultures, we find many indicators of a sober realism about death. Sometimes we even find an excess or morbid preoccupation with death.[19] Beginning with the period of the French revolution and the enlightenment, we find in human thought an increasingly optimistic and often naive viewpoint on life and death. One scholar remarks that there are many persons who probably expect that next month's *Reader's Digest* will carry the headline story that death has been conquered forever.[20] This utopianism has been stimulated by the incredible successes which medicine has in fact experienced over the past century.

Part of this utopianism is a fear of death and a desire to avoid dealing with death at all costs. Many elements in our society (notably including entertainment media and advertising) spend time deemphasizing death, and instead emphasizing realities such as youth, beauty, physical prowess, and sexual gratification. The result is that both health care providers and those seeking health care can slip uncritically into a "do everything possible" mentality. This mentality is applied both to individual patients and to the health care system as a whole (in terms of research priorities, etc.). With this perspective, the fact that none of us can avoid death is overlooked. The cost of developing medical technologies is also overlooked, as is the negative impact of high medical expenditures on our ability to enhance the human good in areas such as education, housing, and the arts. Because this question of our attitude toward death has so many religious and moral overtones, it will be a major focus in our third and fourth chapters.

Insufficient Emphasis on Preventive Medicine

The last point to be mentioned in our analysis of factors which drive up the cost of health care has to do with the relative lack of success which our health care system has had in emphasizing preventive health care measures. It is clear that human health depends to a great degree on good health habits such as adequate rest, proper nutrition, and regular exercise, on environmental factors such as clean water and clear air, and on avoidance of risky behaviors such as alcohol and drug abuse. But in many ways our health care system seems to focus on helping people once they get sick, rather than focusing on the less costly steps which might help people stay healthy in the first place. There have been some important U.S. successes in terms of preventive medicine (dentistry is a good example), and we must acknowledge that some people will get seriously sick and need major care even if they have good health habits. But the lack of emphasis on preventive medicine contributes to the high cost of our health care system. Even in terms of basic steps like polio vaccinations, the U.S. has a disturbingly low immunization rate when compared to some other countries.[21]

One prominent example of the underemphasis in the United States on preventive medicine stems from the area of prenatal care.

Much of the money we spend on neonatal intensive care could be saved if we provided proper prenatal care to poor mothers. Recently neonatal intensive care in New York City has cost about $190 million per year or nearly a tenth of the $2.2 billion annual budget of New York's Health and Hospitals Corporation.[22]

The cost issue and the prevention issue can relate to each other in a vicious cycle. Because all health care is costly, poor people can be afraid to seek basic health care which will often involve some preventive measures or measures to keep existing conditions from getting worse. The result is that when poor people finally do seek health care they are often very sick, even desperately sick. In the end their care may end up being much more expensive. Without doubt, any effort to reform U.S. health care will need to involve a significantly increased emphasis on preventive care.

STRESSES IN THE HEALTH CARE SYSTEM

In the previous two sections of this chapter we have looked at the uninsured and at major reasons for the high cost of health care. As part of the picture of the problems of health care delivery in the U.S., it must also be noted that the issues mentioned above have created many very difficult points of stress for our health care delivery system. In this section we will consider six major points of stress: charity and uncompensated care, poorly focused cost shifting, the growth of covert rationing, pressures on emergency medicine, cultural pressures, and the AIDS crisis.

Charity and Uncompensated Care

For centuries doctors and health care institutions have provided charity care to needy patients. Wonderful stories of heroism and generosity can be told about such charity care, and for a long time almost all the health care needs of the poor were able to be met through this kind of charity. Older doctors occasionally write with a wistful tone about the good old days when doctors spent a half day (or some other portion of their time) each week giving free care to those who could not pay.[23] One might wish that those good old days could return and that the medical charity system of the past could meet our needs today.

It would of course be naive to think that earlier approaches to charity care could be completely effective in our era in which health care is so expensive. But the fact remains that health care profession-

als and health care institutions still experience a strong sense of responsibility toward those who cannot pay for their care. A survey
estimates that in 1988, U.S. doctors gave patients more than $6 billion
dollars worth of uncompensated care, and a similar survey for 1989
estimates that health care institutions gave patients more than $11
billion worth of uncompensated care.[24] The surveys use the general
term "uncompensated care" since health care providers determine
their uncollected income by adding two main categories: the charity
category which covers expenses for patients who are known from the
outset to be unable to pay, and the bad debts category which covers
expenses for patients who never paid their bills even though they
were originally thought to be able to do so. But whatever the language, the surveys suggest that our health care system is giving away a
vast amount of free care, perhaps a total of about $17 billion annually.

These figures for uncompensated care have risen sharply over
the past decade, with health care institutions now giving about $7
billion dollars more for uncompensated care than they did in 1980.
There is no doubt that most of our health care institutions are stretch-
ing themselves to meet the growing crisis in the delivery of health
care. While Roman Catholic health care centers have always had a
strong commitment to charity care, many Roman Catholic institutions
have begun to reflect more explicitly on their role as givers of uncompensated care. The Catholic Health Association has prepared a study
text known as the *Social Accountability Budget.*[25] This text has been the
basis for a renewed awareness about charity care in many Catholic
institutions.

Part of the reason for the high level of uncompensated care can
be found in the changes initiated in the Medicare system during the
Reagan years. Mr. Reagan's administration established a new method
of Medicare payment which is known by the acronym DRG (diagnosis
related groupings). In the DRG system, there are about 460 different
ways to be sick, and for each way to be sick there is a set amount which
Medicare will pay, no matter how much it actually costs to care for a
given patient. Such a system creates incentives for hospitals to dis-
charge patients as quickly as possible, and it also means that hospitals
may have to take losses on patients whose care costs more than the
DRG will pay.

In fairness to the Reagan approach, at its beginning the DRG
payment method did push health care institutions to find more efficient ways to treat many types of patients. It was also true that, in the
first few years of the DRG system, some health care institutions found
ways to offer more uncompensated care than they had previously

delivered. However, as the years have passed, the government has tended to raise its reimbursements for the different DRGs more slowly than the actual costs of care have risen. So even those facets of DRGs which showed early promise are less present today.

Whatever the merits or demerits of the DRG system, an analysis of the current state of charity care shows that many health care centers are strained to their very limits by today's high load of charity and bad debt cases. The news media all too frequently are reporting cases of "patient dumping," i.e. one health care institution passing on indigent patients to other institutions, because the first institution does not want to take any more patients for whose care it will be uncompensated. Some states are enacting laws to control patient dumping, but there are still some forms of patient dumping which are allowed by law. From the moral viewpoint, it is surely true that many instances of patient dumping are unacceptable. The occurrence of patient dumping is a clear signal that our health care system may be near the breaking point.

Problems Related to Cost Shifting

Hospitals have always been aware that some of their services will be given a higher level of compensation than others. They have known that revenues from their more successful departments can be used to offset costs in other departments which generate less revenue. Even more so, hospitals have known that they can use the revenues generated by their insured patients to offset the cost of caring for indigent patients who have no health care coverage. These practices are known as cost shifting, and they have long been a standard part of health care financing. Because of the usefulness of cost shifting, hospitals tend to be concerned that they have a reasonable mix of private patients who have insurance and service patients for whom no coverage may be available.[26]

What has happened in recent years, however, is that, as health care expenses have increased, the need for cost shifting has gotten greater and greater, with the result that cost shifting procedures are much less focused and putting ever greater stress on the health care delivery system as a whole. New reimbursement schemes for private patients (such as prospective payments, discounts for using certain physicians, etc.) have made cost shifting less and less feasible. We are at or near the point when traditional cost shifting procedures will be unable to meet our health care delivery needs as a society.

Part of the problem is that our health care delivery system has not been critically reflective on the question of which issues appropriately deserve cost shifting and which do not. It may well be that many aspects of cost shifting should never have existed in the first place. It is clear that substantive health care reform will need to bring about changes in many cost shifting practices.

An issue related to cost shifting has to do with the way in which health insurance companies spread the costs of various health services among the clients they serve. No doubt the focus of health insurance systems is to spread costs among a pool of patients. But are there some health related costs which it is inappropriate to spread among a pool of patients? For example, in some states the cost of having a test tube baby is a mandated insurance benefit, meaning that the cost of a test tube baby is shifted to everyone who is paying for OB-GYN insurance, if not to everyone who is paying for any health insurance. Even if one were uncertain about whether to accept the Catholic Church's clear teaching against test tube babies, it still seems highly doubtful that we should use a cost shifting procedure to pay for test tube babies. Other similar examples might also be given, but the main point is clear: cost shifting and risk spreading practices in health care are not well focused. Problems with these practices are part of our growing overall failure to meet people's health care needs.

Covert or Soft Rationing

As we move further into the heart of this book, the question of health care rationing will become more and more prominent. We live in a finite world, with finite health care resources. In health care and in many other areas of life, we cannot provide all the possible goods which society might desire. In view of our limits, can we choose not to provide some potentially beneficial health treatments because there are other health treatments and other social goods which are even more beneficial? The depths of this major question will be explored later.

However, when some people first hear the rationing question, their instinctive response is to say something like: "Oh, no. We can't have health care rationing. We can't ever withhold any beneficial treatment from any patient!" As this instinctive comment implies, our current health care system never describes itself as offering health care on a rationed basis. It must be admitted, however, that there is already a great deal of covert rationing in today's health care delivery system. Statistics show that a number of expensive medical procedures are significantly more likely to be made available to rich patients than to poor patients. Due to the pressures of high costs, stretched revenues, and large charity demands, our health care system has become in many respects a system of secret rationing. Some authors see this as one of the most troubling aspects of health care delivery today.[27]

Later, in a more detailed analysis, I will argue that a carefully managed and sensitive system of health care rationing could be moral under certain circumstances. But from the outset it seems clear that covert rationing based on the economic status of patients is not a moral option. Instead, the health care system's covert resort to health care rationing is just one more sign that our current approach to health care delivery is not working.

Emergency Rooms and the Health Care System

To get a graphic picture of the state of health care delivery today, one only needs to take a look at the character of many hospital emergency rooms. Because so many persons are without health care insurance and without a primary care physician, there is a whole class of persons for whom hospital emergency rooms are their primary health center. Such persons cannot go anywhere else for health care; when they get sick they go to the emergency room, even if they are not sick enough to need the kind of care which emergency rooms are equipped to offer. Many modern emergency rooms have responded wonderfully to the difficult task of serving as a back-up for an inadequate health care system. Many dedicated physicians and nurses work in such emergency rooms. But the fact remains that in many ways today's emergency rooms are a prime symbol of all the pressures facing our health care delivery system. All too often, especially in inner city emergency rooms in large urban areas, the patient mix will include people who are car accident victims, persons suffering cardiac arrest, drug addicts, homeless persons who need care for minor ailments such as colds, and other uninsured persons who need routine care. Without changes to make health care more accessible to all, the character of today's emergency rooms is only likely to worsen.

Caring for Persons with AIDS

It would have been possible to simply list AIDS along with all the other factors which make health care cost so much. The cost for research on the disease and the cost of caring for AIDS patients is already very high and will only get higher as more of the million or so Americans who are HIV positive actually become AIDS patients over the years ahead. Without doubt the total cost for AIDS will be many billions of dollars. Some health experts think that a cure for AIDS is still a long way off, but that in the meantime techniques for caring for AIDS patients will get better and better. The result may well be that, at least for a period of time in the years ahead, numbers of AIDS patients will have more of a chronic disease than a disease which will be fatal over a fairly short term. If so, the costs for long term care of AIDS patients will become more and more of a factor.

But in spite of all these direct financial costs, it seems better to understand AIDS as creating stresses for our health care system in many different ways, not simply in financial terms. For one thing, AIDS patients usually die at a fairly young age, so that the health care delivery system can find it hard to face up to their death. In addition, the fact that many AIDS patients are drug abusers or homosexual persons means that caregivers often need special attitudinal education to help them deal well with AIDS patients. Also, there is a great need for education about the nature of AIDS, about the ways in which it is transmitted, etc. Such education is needed for both caregivers and for the public in general. Finally there is the whole matter of testing to see if someone (either a patient or a caregiver) is HIV positive. Voluntary testing of high risk groups and suitable structures to monitor their health and determine acceptable practice standards for HIV positive caregivers are needed. But large scale mandatory testing of patients and the public disclosure of the HIV status of all health-care workers do not seem indicated, either morally or economically, even if such approaches are politically attractive.

Along with each of these stress points related to AIDS, there are additional financial costs. A detailed analysis of these stress points (and of other related issues which we have not mentioned) would go beyond the scope of this book. The point here is simple. AIDS is creating a great many problems for our already overburdened health system. Careful reflection is called for to be sure that all the moral issues related to AIDS are properly addressed.[28]

Cultural Perspectives and Health Care Delivery

Another factor which creates pressure on our health care delivery system today is the rapidly expanding multicultural character of the U.S. population. In addition to the long-standing African-American population, more and more people in the U.S. are now Hispanics (from various Latino cultures) and Asians. Contemporary political changes in the world may add further to this cultural mix by bringing substantial numbers of Eastern Europeans and persons from the Middle East into our country.

This multiculturalism is important in the health care context because persons from different cultures will often understand and describe medical symptoms differently than Anglo-Americans. To be effective in multicultural health care delivery, our health care system will need to be sure that more and more caregivers understand not only different languages but also different cultural approaches to health care. The cost of expanding multicultural awareness in the delivery of health care will be high, but a failure to do so could be even more costly in the long run.[29]

One of my most memorable experiences of ethics in health care was being consulted by a hospital on how to proceed in dealing with a young woman who had been diagnosed as carrying an anencephalic baby. While I was thinking about the general ethical principles which might apply in this case, it quickly became clear that the underlying problem was that the hospital in question had no one who was sufficiently fluent in the young woman's language to explain to her what it meant that her baby was anencephalic. This took place many years ago, and I am sure it would not happen in the same hospital today. But the larger challenge and cost of multicultural health care continues to be very much with us.

STRESS ON THE U.S. ECONOMY
AND GROWING PUBLIC FRUSTRATION
WITH HEALTH CARE

The last few paragraphs have focused on some of the ways in which our health care system is stressed near or to its breaking point by our current approach to health care delivery. But we need also to note that the difficulties of our health system touch much more than health care alone. Almost everything in American life, especially in American economic life, seems to be affected by the high cost of health care. Economists tell us that the U.S. is now spending about 13% of its gross national product (GNP) on health care.[30] This percentage of GNP is up by 4–5% over the past decade, and this percentage is about half again as large as the percentage of GNP spent on health care in most other industrialized countries. In addition, it seems clear that if our health care system continues as is, the percent of GNP we spend on health care will keep on rising. Conservative estimates predict that, by the end of the century, an unreformed U.S. health care system will consume 15% of our GNP.[31] But there are estimates such as that of the Kaiser health system which predict that an unchanged health system will be costing the U.S. 22% of its GNP by the year 2000. Even if such a figure is high,[32] there is very grave doubt about the ability of the U.S. economy to keep on sustaining continued increases in the cost of health care.

The high cost of health care means that whatever we pay for (education, housing, etc.) will be more expensive because of the health care costs of the teachers, home builders, etc. Since so many of us are able to focus major economic costs in terms of buying an automobile, it is interesting to ask how much of the cost for a new car goes toward the manufacturer's health care costs. Chrysler chairman Lee Iacocca estimated that in 1988 an average of $700 of the purchase price of every new Chrysler product went toward covering Chrysler's health insurance costs. By 1992 the health care cost for a U.S. built car had reached $1,086.[33] This figure will surely keep on increasing if health care costs continue to rise.

In view of these kinds of figures, it is no surprise that more and more U.S. business executives now think it is essential that we move toward some kind of health care reform. A recent poll showed about two-thirds of corporate executives to be in favor of some type of health care reform.[34] This is interesting since in U.S. history business leaders have tended to oppose government involvement in social programs such as support for health care. But in recent years, the U.S. business community has developed a very important perspective on the whole issue: How can the U.S. produce products which will compete with products from elsewhere in the world, if we keep on trying to pay for such a costly and inefficient health care delivery system? Business leaders worry that the U.S. will face economic collapse as a nation unless it comes up with a better health care system.

It is important to focus on these concerns about health care and the economic capacity of the U.S. But there are many other issues in terms of how health care costs relate to the whole character of our society. For a long time the U.S. spent about as much each year on education as it did on health care. We now spend about twice as much on health care as on education, and these cost increases in health care have made it harder and harder for governments and private groups in the U.S. to fund education. Many worry that our education system may be nearing the point of collapse in terms of the ability to provide a good quality education to most young people. Similar concerns can be raised about other areas of life.

In general, I think it can be said that people as a whole have caught on to the problems of health care and know that some kind of change will be necessary between now and the end of the century. Very many Americans will say that they personally have had good health care, but, as I mentioned in the Introduction, only about 10% of persons in the U.S. will say that our health care system is just fine as is or only in need of minor changes. By comparison, about 60% of Canadians will say that their health care system is fine as it stands or only needs minor adjustments.[35] Even though this figure shows a large number of Canadians who are not satisfied with their system, the percentage of satisfied Canadians is dramatically higher than in the U.S. percentage. We will have more to say about the Canadian system in the next chapter.

If it is true that many Americans have personally had good health care, why is it that so many think that the U.S. system needs major changes? In part, the answer is that even those who have been treated well in the U.S. have experienced long waits, confusing billing, uninsured family and friends, inefficient arrangement of services, etc. In part, too, I think it can be argued that many in the U.S. are at least intuitively experiencing the larger concerns which have been explicitly cited by the business community and other leaders. All in all, it is clear that this chapter's concerns about health care go beyond health care itself. The entire quality of life in the U.S. is being placed at risk by the problems of our health care system.

In one sense, I hope this chapter has not been too depressing, since health care in the U.S. does have many proud accomplishments. But the problems in U.S. health care are very real, and it was essential for this book to summarize the problems so as to set the context for our project of theological/moral reflection on potential new directions for U.S. health care.

Chapter 2

OTHER OPTIONS
AND OTHER COUNTRIES

As was just mentioned, the main purpose of this book will be to move on to some theological and moral reflections on health care delivery. However, besides the just completed review of U.S. health care delivery today, we need a brief description of the major options for change which are currently being proposed for the U.S. health care system as a whole. We also need to examine the systems of health care delivery which have been adopted in other countries, especially countries with economies similar to that in the U.S. Likewise, we will need to consider health reform initiatives which states such as Vermont and Oregon have recently enacted into law. Our theological/moral reflections will only be meaningful if we have established a solid understanding of what some of the concretely viable reform possibilities are. Such a solid understanding of the possibilities is the goal of this chapter. The chapter will be divided into four sections. First, we shall discuss some of the proposals for health care reform which have been suggested in the United States over the past quarter century or so. Many of these earlier proposals focused on purely private reforms, i.e. reforms from within the health care delivery system involving little or no legislative change. Second, we shall look at several types of current legislative proposals which seek to bring about national reform of the U.S. health care delivery system. Third, we will look at health care delivery in other countries, especially in Canada and Great Britain. Finally, we will consider changes in health care delivery which have recently occurred or been proposed in some individual American states.

SOME EARLIER PROPOSALS FOR HEALTH CARE REFORM

Almost as soon as people began to be aware of the need for changes in the delivery of health care, calls for private health care reform began to surface. Many experts today think that the problems with health care delivery are too complex to be resolved by private action alone. Still, there are some important health care reforms which have taken place through private actions. Future planning for health care reform needs to attend to the possibilities for private change and to learn from the successes which have taken place on this basis. Some of these successes may be able to be incorporated into a comprehensive national plan for health care reform.

The HMOs or health maintenance organizations to which we alluded in the last chapter are probably the paradigmatic example of private sector change in the delivery of health care. HMOs took their origin under the leadership of the industrialist Henry J. Kaiser who in the late 1930s needed to find a way to provide health care for the construction workers who were building the Grand Coulee Dam. During the Second World War, the Kaiser health plan quickly spread to Kaiser steel mills and shipyards on the west coast. After the war the plan became available to non-Kaiser employees in the west and in Hawaii. The main concept behind the HMO is that those enrolled in an HMO pay an annual fee (often called a capitation fee) to cover all medical care rather than being billed and dealing with insurers for each health care service which they receive.[1] This approach breaks the fee-for-service psychology which we discussed in the last chapter. Many persons pay an annual maintenance fee for their computers or other types of property. The HMO treats health care costs in a somewhat similar fashion.

In some HMOs, the doctors remain self-employed and receive payment from the HMO for their services. But in other, stronger HMOs, the doctors are salaried employees of the HMO. Because they collect fixed annual fees, HMOs have an incentive to keep the costs down by avoiding unnecessary testing, unnecessary admissions to hospitals, etc. The HMO also has the incentive of trying to provide quality medical care so as to attract more patients. In recent years, HMOs have grown popular in all parts of the U.S. Many employers now offer their employees an HMO option at a lower cost than a traditional insurance plan.

Many patients will state that they are very satisfied with the care they receive from an HMO. But there are some complaints too. One common complaint about HMOs is that patients cannot choose their doctors and may be involuntarily moved from doctor to doctor. In many cases this complaint (which can also occur in other health care settings) is unfounded, but it remains a worry for some. Another point of concern is that some (not all) HMOs have a rather high rate of patient turnover. This may suggest that some HMOs use aggressive marketing strategies to enroll new patients but fail later on to provide as strong a quality of care as some patients desire. In addition, HMOs, like insurance companies, can be tempted to market themselves to low risk patients while avoiding the enrollment of higher risk patients. Sensitive employers are often able to discover and establish relationships with those local HMOs which have the best reputations.

A more recent private sector reform is the preferred provider organization (PPO). In a PPO set up, the employers' insurance companies ask physicians (who remain self-employed) to meet certain standards in terms of discounted charges, etc. If a physician agrees to meet the PPO's standards, patients using this physician are able to pay a lower insurance rate. PPOs are often able to enroll hundreds and even thousands of physicians in a local area, meaning that patients are able to choose from a wide spectrum of physicians. As with HMOs, many employers now make PPO options available to their employees. PPOs are not perfect since patients may not always be able to get the doctor they want or the service they want. But PPOs are a significant move toward a more effective and efficient management of health care.

Another interesting and complex change in the delivery of health care has been the development of drive-in clinics and rapid health care centers. In an age when many people lack access to a primary care physician (because of travel, lack of insurance, etc.), such centers can provide easy access to simple care needs and thus take the pressure off hospital emergency rooms. The easy convenience of such centers reminds me of the fast food industry.

Caution is needed in assessing the role of these drive-in clinics and related health services. Some of them seem to have been founded largely as money-making operations, without enough attention to true quality care. Nonetheless, such centers, if managed with a commitment to quality care and ethical standards, may have the potential to make simple health services more readily accessible at a lower cost. Obviously, such centers will never be able to provide for more complex health care needs.

Health care providers such as hospitals and nursing homes have also been able to develop some important reforms on a private basis. Better internal management has in many places helped to keep costs down. Hospital structures such as utilization review (to help avoid the furnishing of unnecessary services) and quality assurance (to be sure that appropriate care is being rendered) have been particularly helpful in the achievement of efficient quality care. The development of one-day surgery centers has been both cost effective and (sometimes) good for patients.

In the same context, many health care institutions have recently moved into joint ventures with other health care providers. In such joint ventures, a hospital may link up with a nearby OB clinic, a nearby nursing home, a group of physicians, etc., enabling all of the partners in the joint venture to offer a wider range of health care services. While it is not possible to offer a complete treatment of joint ventures in this book, I would like to offer three comments.[2]

First, it is understandable that physicians would want to be a part of joint ventures, and in the past some physicians became involved in joint ventures for very laudatory reasons. One thinks for instance of the immigrant groups and racial minorities in the U.S. who had real trouble in attaining quality care until doctors from these groups were able to found hospitals, clinics, etc. On the other hand, joint ventures as they exist today often present doctors with very difficult conflicts of interest. If a doctor is an owner or part owner of a medical service, why does he or she refer a patient to that service? For the sake of more business for the service, or because of the true need of the patient? Such questions may make Catholic hospitals wonder whether they should engage in any joint ventures with doctors, and some experts think that all doctor involvement in joint ventures should be banned because of this kind of problem. Others would accept doctor involvement in joint ventures, but only with very careful controls such as full disclosure and non-ability to refer one's own patients.

Second, joint ventures can raise some complex problems for Roman Catholic health care centers because the moral standards of a Roman Catholic center may not be shared by a prospective joint venturer. For instance, what if the partner with the Catholic center wants to provide contraception devices or surgical sterilization? Later in the book we will be talking about the theme of material cooperation which can help set a framework out of which Catholic health care facilities might approach joint venture questions.

Third, we live in an age in which many people find health care services both divided and confusing. If the proper ethical framework can be established, joint ventures would have the potential for helping people's health care needs be met in a more integrated fashion. We will look at this issue further when we consider the shape of health care reform in Chapter 8.

The questions of physician distribution and specialization are often cited as areas for health care reform. It is suggested for instance that procedures for physician licensure might be arranged to make rural and inner city practices more attractive to doctors. Similarly, scholarship monies for attendance at medical schools could be tied to an early period of medical service in an area where doctors are scarce. Scholarship monies could also be tied to needed areas of specialty such as family medicine. Some of the proposals along these lines move beyond the areas of private action (e.g. state laws which would limit the number of doctor's licenses available in a given area), but the proposed changes are often seen as constructive possibilities for health care reform.

In the late 1970s and the early 1980s, the debate about health care reform moved from the private initiatives mentioned above to more concern about health care reform through public sector activity. In terms of public policy changes, one of the first issues to come to the fore was the question of a national program of catastrophic health insurance, i.e. insurance to pay for the cost of illness situations which are so expensive that the cost of the illness will wipe out the life savings of most individuals and families. Both the Carter and the Reagan administrations proposed legislation to provide catastrophic health insurance, and some coverage of catastrophic illness for low income uninsured persons did become law in the Reagan years.[3]

As the very term implies, catastrophic illness can be a human disaster for many families, and a national insurance program for catastrophic illness seems very reasonable. It is important to remember, however, that programs to insure some catastrophic illnesses are only a drop in the bucket in terms of the overall problem of the quarter of the U.S. population which is uninsured or underinsured. Some of the proposals on catastrophic insurance actually reduced other kinds of health care coverage, meaning that the early proposals on catastrophic coverage were in some ways a politically attractive front for failing to do more to provide for people's wider health care needs.[4] Add to all this the fact that with ever-growing costs, almost any serious illness can be said to be financially catastrophic for many persons. Hence it is clear that the U.S. cannot solve its overall health care delivery problems by providing coverage for a few key catastrophic illnesses.

To sum up, the past twenty-five years saw the development of a number of important initiatives to help reform health care delivery. Many of these initiatives called for private sector action, but some of them did advocate changes in public policy. These earlier initiatives raised interesting approaches along with some new problems. In general, these earlier initiatives can be a useful learning experience for us as we face health care reform today. Very few people, however, would claim that these earlier initiatives are adequate to address today's problems in the area of just health care delivery. Thus we must move on to consider the current proposals for health care reform.

CURRENT PROPOSALS FOR NATIONWIDE REFORM OF THE U.S. HEALTH CARE DELIVERY SYSTEM

I turn to the area of current proposals for U.S. health care reform with some fear and trepidation, because there is so much material to assess in terms of current health care reform proposals. By the middle of 1991 there were more than a dozen serious proposals for health care reform which had been put together by foundations, public interest groups, research groups, congressional and senatorial staffs, etc. These serious proposals alone make for a fascinating study. But since the middle of 1991, there has been an enormous surge of public interest in the topic of health care reform. Almost every day one reads in the newspapers about new proposals for health care reform or at least about new variations on the existing proposals. The large and surprising electoral victory of health care reform advocate Sen. Harris Wofford in the special Pennsylvania senate race was in many ways a signal event which has served to crystalize national attention on health care reform.

It obviously would be impossible to describe each proposal for health care reform in detail. Instead, this section will divide the national proposals for health care reform into five main categories. There will be a description of each category and a summary of some of the specific proposals which belong to each category. The five categories of proposals are: first, proposals which limit themselves to tax reforms which will enhance access to the private U.S. delivery system; second, universal access proposals which retain the present tripartite coverage system (i.e. Medicare, Medicaid and private insurance); third, universal access proposals which retain a combination of public coverage and private, employment-based coverage, but with more substantive changes in the public coverage (including the elimination of Medicaid); fourth, proposals which move toward a single public payer approach to health care insurance, but with a continued role for a multiplicity of private insurance carriers; fifth, proposals for a true single payer national health insurance system.

Two preliminary comments are in order. First, the fivefold categorization of the proposals will serve as a basis for understanding and comparing many of the current proposals for health care reform. But

in actual fact, some of the specific proposals belong more purely under one of the five categories, while other proposals may tend to
overlap the categories. Every typological analysis has its limitations,
but my judgment is that a division of the proposals into categories will
lead to a better assessment of many of today's reform proposals. In
terms of an organizing rationale, the five categorizations will move
from proposals which suggest relatively less change to proposals
which call for more extensive reforms.

The second preliminary comment relates to the popular media's
increasingly frequent use of the term "play or pay" as a descriptor for
a major set of health reform proposals. The idea behind this term is
that health care reform laws should either make employers provide
health insurance for their employees (i.e. to "play") or cause employers to be taxed ("pay") so that the tax monies can be used to cover the
employees who are not insured through their work. In the list of five
categories, both categories two and three contain some "play or pay"
proposals. As this implies, there are some important differences
among the play or pay proposals. Thus I have not chosen to use play
or pay as a main category in my summary of the current proposals for
health care reform.

Proposals Limited to Tax Reforms To Enhance
Access to the Private U.S. Health System

When we think about the U.S. government's role in the delivery
of health care we very quickly begin to think about specific government programs such as Medicare and Medicaid. In actual fact the U.S.
government helped facilitate access to health care long before Medicare and Medicaid existed. The government's earlier and still continuing policy for access takes place through the tax system, i.e. through
tax policies which permit measures such as the itemized deduction of
health care expenses.

Thus it is no surprise that one major series of proposals for health
care reform focuses on the use of the tax system as a means of providing more access to health care. The Washington, D.C.-based Heritage
Foundation has been a leader in this kind of thinking with its proposal
that significant tax credits be made available to help people pay for
the cost of health care.[5] Other similar suggestions have been made
about special tax policies which would make it easier for small businesses to purchase health insurance for their employees. Still other
suggestions of this same type are beginning to emerge, and it will be
important to understand the various tax reform proposals which are

intended to enhance access to health care. It seems that some advocates of tax credits, etc., are so confident in these approaches that they believe that in time measures like tax credits will even be able to replace Medicare and Medicaid.

No doubt tax credits would enable some people to purchase health insurance. However, I think there are very serious concerns about the concept of changing tax laws to enhance access to health care reform. For instance, while such tax changes would help some of the thirty-seven million people without health insurance, it seems that such changes would still leave many persons with no health insurance. Even more fundamentally, the tax reform approach in no way addresses the fact that our health care delivery system seems to be seriously flawed and grossly inefficient. From this perspective, all that tax credits will do is to pump more money into an already very troubled health system. Along the same lines, tax credits offer no leadership to help the U.S. decide what its true priorities ought to be in health care. The tax credit approach trusts the free market approach to be able to solve all of the health care difficulties of the U.S. Valuable as the free market is for the economy in general, there are growing concerns that in health care a market economy is a significant cause of many of the current problems, such as the inability of persons with some health conditions to buy insurance. Thus a market economy is not likely to be able to redirect the course of U.S. health care, especially if it is the only avenue used to help achieve health care reform. Later we shall see that, while Catholic social teaching has great respect for the free market, it does not believe that a market economy, free of all controls, is able to solve our most complex social problems.

In his January 1992 State of the Union Address (with details in a later follow-up message), President Bush specifically endorsed tax credits of up to $3,750 as a means to health care reform. But the full amount of this tax credit would only be available to those earning less than $7,000, and many persons above that limit are lacking in health care. In addition, health insurance for some families may well cost $6,000 or more, meaning that the top credit of $3,750 would still not enable many poor families to purchase health insurance. Also, it appeared that the Bush proposal would reduce some funding for Medicare and Medicaid, further exacerbating the health care problems faced by the poor and by many older persons. It was hard not to have the impression that the president's proposal was put together quickly and without in-depth thought, due to the growing national demand for health care reform. Even if one were committed to the tax credit strategy, there might still be questions about how well the president's proposal embodies that strategy.

Proposals for Universal Access Which Retain the Present
Tripartite System (Medicare-Medicaid-Private Insurance)

In our second major reform category, we shall consider a group of health care reform proposals which have three goals. First, these proposals want to use tax monies to assure that all poor people have access to health care. Second, these proposals want to create a situation in which all working persons are somehow insured as a result of their employment. Third, these proposals want to accomplish their first and second goals while retaining, at least in large measure, the present tripartite insurance system in which people's health care needs are covered by private insurance, Medicare, or Medicaid, either alone or in some combination with one another. In addition to seeking to provide health insurance for everyone, these proposals also seek to improve both the quality and the efficiency of the care which is delivered through the tripartite system. While they may differ as to specifics, the universal access proposals which use most or all of the tripartite model are basically seeking to repair the present health care system. They are not trying to develop a radically new system.

Here we will survey four of these "fix the system" proposals so as to see some of their different approaches to coverage of the poor, financing, cost management, quality control, etc. The four proposals we will consider are the Kennedy/Waxman plan, the AMA Health Access America Plan, the Consumer Choice Health Plan, and the Proposal of the National Leadership Commission on Health Care.

Perhaps the most paradigmatic example of a reform proposal committed to the tripartite system is the Basic Health Care for All Americans Act, proposed in 1987 by Sen. Edward Kennedy and Rep. Henry Waxman of California.[6] This proposal, which has roots in proposals made by Sen. Kennedy as far back as the mid-1970s, would require employers to cover all full time employees, with employers paying 80% of the cost of health insurance and the employees the other 20%. It would expand the Medicaid program to cover all the poor and the uninsured. Kennedy/Waxman would assure a decent level of benefits, including some mental health services. It would limit any family's out-of-pocket health care expenses to $3,000 per year. Kennedy/Waxman would urge the development of better guidelines for appropriate medical practice and the development of careful cost management strategies.

The Kennedy/Waxman approach is to be praised for its basic goal of providing health care coverage for all Americans. One wonders, however, whether quality care and efficiency of care can be enhanced as long as the present complex administration of health care services remains in place. In addition, while there are estimates of the cost of Kennedy/Waxman for employers ($18–$100 billion per year), the public cost of the program has not yet been estimated. It might also be noted that the Kennedy/Waxman approach is a "play only" model since it requires all employers to provide coverage, rather than giving employers the option of being taxed instead of buying insurance for their employees. (Sen. Kennedy himself has begun to shift his thinking toward a "play or pay" option.)

A second proposal to retain but improve the present system comes from the American Medical Association. Called Health Access America, the AMA plan requires employers to provide insurance for full time employees (to "play"), and it calls for both Medicare and Medicaid reform.[7] The AMA plan wants to put Medicare on a sounder fiscal basis through higher premiums, and it wants employers and employees to contribute throughout working years (instead of after retirement) to an insurance fund to pay for the costs of catastrophic illness. The AMA plan wants Medicaid to cover all poor persons, with greater uniformity in benefits from state to state. The AMA plan realizes that Medicaid reform will be very costly, so it calls for the first steps in reform to be extended to pregnant women and children, something which has already begun to happen through congressional mandate. The AMA plan calls upon states to establish special risk pools for the medically uninsurable and for others who cannot afford individual insurance or qualify for group coverage. The AMA plan also seeks to improve long term care for senior citizens. The AMA estimates that its proposal will cost the federal government $21 billion per year, but it has not produced cost estimates for state governments, local governments, etc. As originally presented, the AMA proposal seemed to offer relatively little in terms of cost containment strategies.

Stanford economist Alain Enthoven has long been interested in health care reform. Together with Richard Kronick, he has proposed the Consumer Choice Health Plan for the 1990s.[8] As with the other two proposals we have considered, Medicare, Medicaid, and private insurance would remain intact, and employers would be required to cover full time workers. Employers would be taxed at 8% for any employees they are not required to cover. (This begins to involve "pay" as well as "play.") A similar tax would apply to the self-employed, retirees, and those uninsured who can afford to pay. These

tax revenues would go to public sponsors who would provide coverage to those who are not covered by Medicare, Medicaid, or
employment-based programs. Those with incomes below 150% of the
poverty line would be fully covered, and no one's out-of-pocket (or
deductible) expenses would be more than 100% of his or her insurance premium (which would be about $3,500 per year for a family).

Two major focus themes of the Enthoven/Kronick proposal are
consumer incentives and managed competition. The Enthoven/
Kronick proposal is very much aware of the inefficiencies and high cost
of our present health care delivery system. The proposal wants to make
employers and employees pay enough of the cost of health care that
these groups will be driven to choose those plans which offer the best
mix of cost efficiency and quality care. Because they pay 80%, employers will be motivated to reward cost effective plans. Employees will
gradually lose some of the tax deductibility which now attaches to their
health benefits, so that they too will want health care plans which are
both fiscally and medically effective. Public sponsors of health care will
be motivated in the same direction. As Enthoven/Kronick see it, the
resulting "managed competition" among health care providers will
lead to widespread private reform of our health care system. It is a
time-honored ethical principle that, as far as possible, social changes
should be brought about without government intervention. But as we
noted earlier, there remains the question of whether non-governmen-
tal approaches to reform can really work. The Enthoven/Kronick proposal assumes that many individuals and many private businesses will
know enough about medicine to exercise effective consumer control
over the delivery of health care services. Granted the enormous complexity of modern health care services, it seems quite uncertain
whether consumer control could be as effective as it is in other segments of the U.S. economy.

The fourth proposal which retains and improves the present tripartite insurance system is the proposal of the National Leadership
Commission on Health Care which was developed by a coalition of
thirty-eight corporations, unions, and foundations.[9] In addition to
some similarities to the three proposals just discussed (such as a
$3,000 limit on out-of-pocket expenses, and a concern for measures
such as preventive care, prenatal care and mental health care), the
National Leadership Commission makes two other significant recommendations. First, it wants each state to set up an uninsured access
(UNAC) program to cover the poor and those receiving acute care
through Medicaid. This step of moving Medicaid administration
more clearly to the states may be more effective than the current

approach, but it still leaves in place three separate health care coverage systems. Second, the Leadership Commission proposes that employers and employees either contribute (in a 75%–25% ratio) to pay for employee health insurance or else be taxed to cover the cost of employee health insurance. The employers would be taxed 9.68% on the first $45,000 of an employee's wages and the employee 2.04%. This plan's tax is not fully progressive since it ends at $45,000, but in this plan the "play or pay" concept is in full flower.

The four proposals we have just reviewed are all to be commended for their basic commitment to assuring that all Americans have access to health care services. They point toward many possible reforms. Critics argue that these programs do not go far enough, and that their commitment to maintaining so much of our present system will ultimately make their proposed reforms ineffective. Dr. William Cleveland of the University of Miami calls these types of programs patches instead of quilts.[10] My intention is not to make final judgments until presenting my theological and moral reflections in Chapters 3 through 6. But it is hard not to agree with Dr. Cleveland's assessment.

Universal Access Proposals with Substantively Changed Public Coverage in Combination with Private, Employment-Based Insurance

In this category we will look at two proposals which continue to combine public programs of health insurance with private, employment-based health insurance. These proposals differ from the previous proposals in that they call for more radical changes in government sponsored health care programs. In particular, these proposals move to replace Medicaid (whose problems we outlined earlier) with new federal and state programs to provide health insurance for the poor.

The first example of such a program comes from Rep. Fortney "Pete" Stark of California whose proposal is called a "MediPlan."[11] In the Stark Mediplan, employers may provide either private insurance or HMO coverage. More first dollar benefits will be required, especially for mothers and children. Nursing home coverage is better, and costs are limited to $2,000 per individual or $3,000 per family. A full subsidy for the cost of health insurance will be available for all Americans at or below 200% of the poverty level. This subsidy will be administered through a new public program similar to Medicare, thereby eliminating the state-to-state unevenness of the Medicaid program. Stark's program includes a 4% tax on personal and corporate incomes over $16,000 per year. The estimate is that Stark's program will eventually cost the U.S. government $120 billion per year. Stark's approach does have the honest realism of admitting that taxes will be necessary and that federal costs for reform will be high. Stark does make some recommendations to help manage costs, including prospective payment systems for hospitals and nursing homes. On the whole the Stark plan calls for some very substantial changes in the delivery of health care. At the same time, the plan does retain the potentially complex combination of private, employment-based insurance with a federally managed health insurance program. In addition, some critics worry that strategies such as prospective payment will result in health care decisions being made for budgetary reasons instead of from an assessment of genuine patient needs.

The proposal of the U.S. Bipartisan Commission on Comprehensive Health Care is another important proposal which wants to reform U.S. health care delivery while retaining the current system of private insurance.[12] The Bipartisan Commission, created by the U.S. Congress, is usually called the Pepper Commission. It is chaired by Sen. John D. Rockefeller IV of West Virginia. The Pepper Commission calls for some very significant changes in the delivery of health care. It clearly calls for universal coverage for all Americans. It calls for a new federal program similar to Medicare to replace Medicaid and provide care for the poor. Its proposed coverages are similar to those of the Kennedy/Waxman proposal. It estimates its cost to be $66 billion per year, and it recommends a progressive financing system, but without being specific.

What is particularly interesting about the Pepper Commission is its insistence on the development of strong national standards to assure that all people are receiving good quality care.[13] Similarly, the Pepper Commission has some important suggestions for cost containment, including malpractice reforms, managed care, and the insistence that its new federal program for the poor be administered like Medicare rather than like Medicaid. Sen. Rockefeller seems thoroughly knowledgeable about the Commission's agenda, and he may become a significant national leader for health care reform.

Along with all its calls for reform, the Pepper Commission is very explicit in its conservative judgment that the U.S. must retain a mix of private, employer-based insurance along with federal programs to provide for the aged and the poor.[14] This fact leads Dr. Cleveland to describe the Pepper Commission proposals as another patch instead of a radical call for change,[15] even though the Pepper Commission calls for many significant reforms in the health care system.

*Programs Calling for Unified National Financing
with Administration by Private Insurers*

The proposals discussed in the last two sections all called for a combination of private employment-based insurance and public programs of health insurance. The two proposals we are now going to consider move toward the idea of a single national plan for financing all patients. This plan will be administered by the states. Private insurors may still exist, with their health coverage plans to be approved by each state. The funding for each person will come from the unified health care financing system.

The first example of this concept of unified government financing along with the private administration of insurance is the Health Security Partnership which has been proposed by Rashi Fein of the Harvard Medical School.[16] The key concept behind the Health Security Partnership is that the federal and state governments must work together to provide health insurance for all Americans. The role of the federal government will be to set fundamental national standards for what must be covered, to take steps to enhance the quality and efficiency of health care delivery, and to provide the states with substantial financial support for their individual health care programs.

The states, as partners with the federal government, will be expected to meet the federal standards so as to receive federal funding. For example, the states will have to show that at least 95% of their citizens have health insurance. Once the states have met the federal standards, they will have quite a bit of flexibility as to how they provide coverage. They may continue to use private insurors to administer their programs, using strategies like fixed budgets, fee schedules, and prospective payment to assure efficient delivery of health care services. They may choose to collect insurance premiums from employers, and they may enact appropriate taxes to help meet the needs of their programs. The key point is that there would be a unified flow of all sources of health care funding into a state agency. This would enable better management of health costs and it would mean that any insurance companies used by the states would be unable to discriminate between public and privately funded patients.

One of the more unique aspects of the Health Security Partnership proposal is its emphasis on the importance of leaving a good deal of latitude in the hands of each state. Rashi Fein is aware of regional differences in the U.S., and he thinks it is good for the states to be able to use different approaches. Some states may wish to eliminate private insurance carriers, some may wish to eliminate employment-based premiums in favor of taxes, etc. The idea is that as long as basic federal standards are met, each state should be able to do what works best for it. In this context, Fein quotes Justice Louis Brandeis' notion that the state ought to serve as the nation's experimental laboratories.[17]

The Health USA Act of 1991 is a second example of a health care reform program which takes a unified approach to funding while leaving a role for private insurors. The Health USA Act has been proposed by Sen. Robert Kerrey of Nebraska.[18] Sen. Kerrey's proposal has three main goals: cost containment, universal access to health care, and single payer financing independent of employment. The Health USA Act would create a National Health Care Commission of eight members to set guidelines for the states, establish national standards for quality care and cost management, set priorities for national and regional health needs, etc. State programs (or programs sponsored by groups of states) would need to meet the basic requirements of the National Commission. Every person would be insured and minimum benefits would include hospital care, physician services, tests, preventive care, prescriptions, and mental health services.

At the level of financing there would be national and state health care budgets, with federal funds flowing to the states. In each state there would be a single payer system, and employment-based health insurance would be eliminated. (Note that this differs from the Health Security Partnership which has a single financing system, but leaves the states with the option of collecting employment-based insurance premiums.) Sen. Kerrey argues that his type of single payment plan will be administratively simpler and therefore more cost effective. The states could choose to administer their own programs, or, more likely, the states could engage a number of competing private insurors to administer their health programs. Individuals who live near other states could get their care in those states, an important point in rural areas.

The existing sources of health care funding (Medicare, Medicaid) will be applied to the new program. New sources of funding include a 5% payroll tax (80% of this to be paid by the employer), a 2% tax increase on non-wage income, a 33% top income tax bracket, a 10% increase in corporate income tax, excise taxes on products like alcohol and tobacco, and an increased tax on Social Security benefits. Individuals will have to pay an annual deductible and a 20% copayment with a cost limit of $2,000 per year for a family of three or more.

Sen. Kerrey contracted with an independent financial analysis firm, which argues that his plan can save the U.S. $150 billion in health care costs over the next five years, due to its unified administration, cost containment incentives, etc. The firm says that the plan would save the average employer $77 per employee per year and that the average Nebraska family would spend $500 per year less on health care under the Health USA Act.[19] Further study is needed to verify these claims, but the potential of a unified system to save money is surely an important aspect in the debate about more just systems of health care delivery. On the whole the Kerrey plan calls for a great deal of reform, but it does leave the private insurance industry in place. One recent report states that more than a million people in the U.S. have jobs related to the processing of health care claims.[20] This makes it hard not to wonder whether we may need something more efficient than a multiplicity of private insurance carriers.

Proposals for True Single Payer National Health Insurance

The final two proposals we will discuss call for the elimination of the competitive private health insurance industry, and for the establishment of a national health insurance system to be administered by the states. These proposals are more sweeping than any we have so far discussed. These proposals are also rather similar to the Canadian health care system which we will be considering shortly.

The first proposal calling for a national insurance system is the Physicians for a National Health Program Proposal.[21] The Physicians for a National Health Program is based at the Center for National Health Program Studies, Cambridge Hospital-Harvard Medical School. The proposal was generated by a writing committee of thirty physicians chaired by Drs. David Himmelstein and Steffie Woolhandler. It has been signed by more than 400 doctors from throughout the U.S., who represent virtually all fields of medical practice.

After beginning with a statement of frustration about the current U.S. health care system, the Physicians' Proposal explicitly calls for the replacement of Medicare, Medicaid, and private insurance with a single public insurance plan to cover all necessary medical services, dental services, prescription drugs, preventive health care, and public health measures. Patients would pay neither copayments nor deductibles. The Physicians' Proposal, unlike other proposals we have seen, is convinced that copayments and deductibles can threaten poor people's health, and that they are not effective in reducing health care cost.[22]

Hospitals would receive an annual lump sum prospective payment from the national health fund, based on past performance, projected changes in service, etc. Each state would have an agency to determine the size of this payment. Physicians would be paid by billing the national health program for each service rendered to a patient. A negotiated fee schedule would be in place and physicians could not charge more than the scheduled fee. Group practices, HMOs, etc., could choose to be paid an annual capitation fee for each patient they serve. The tax mechanisms to be used would include the sources of current Medicare and Medicaid funding, taxes on employers (to take the place of current private health plans) and other taxes to make up for people's out-of-pocket health costs (which will cease to exist).

Perhaps the most crucial aspect of the Physicians' Proposal is its call to eliminate private insurance. The proposal states that there are more than 1,500 private health insurers in the U.S., and that their administrative costs account for 8% of the cost of health care whereas Medicare's administrative cost is only about 3%.[23] The proposal argues that the elimination of private insurance (along with other measures like better health planning and care for the poor before they become very sick and thus very costly to care for) will enable the U.S. to insure all Americans without spending more money than we currently spend as a nation for health care. Companies which are already providing good health insurance for employees will actually save money. It is estimated for example that a company like Chrysler will see its per capita health care expenses move from $5,300 to $1,600.

The second proposal for a national health insurance program is the Universal Health Care Act of 1991, which has been introduced by Congressman Marty Russo of Illinois.[24] Mr. Russo's bill is jointly sponsored by twenty-five other members of Congress, and endorsed by a number of labor unions and other organizations including, not coincidentally, the Physicians for a National Health Program.

The fundamental structure of the Russo bill is essentially the same as the proposal of the Physicians for a National Health Program, but the Russo bill offers more specifics on the administration, financing, and cost for a national health insurance program. Russo clearly specifies that at the national level the program would be administered by the Department of Health and Human Services. The states could administer the program themselves or they could contract with one (only one) private firm to handle the processing of claims. Russo calls for a 6% tax on employers (to replace former insurance premiums), a 4% increase in corporate taxes, a top rate of 38% for federal income tax (for incomes above $200,000), a long term care premium for the elderly increased by $25 over the current Medicare Part B premium, and the making of 85% of Social Security benefits into taxable income.

No doubt the specifics of some of these increases would need to be renegotiated if the bill should ever move toward becoming law.

The Russo bill analyzes health care costs for most major groups in our society: business, the elderly, the non-elderly, charitable groups, state and local governments, and the federal government. The analysis claims that the U.S. as a whole would have spent $40 billion less on health care in 1989 if the Russo bill had then been in effect. The only one of these major groups to have spent more in 1989 would have been business. But even this effect would largely have been on businesses which were not providing health care benefits. Russo states that all businesses will eventually save money because his bill will reduce future increases in health care spending.

Russo acknowledges that his bill does not have all the answers and that many specifics of health care reform still need to be worked out. But the case that a unified health insurance system can save money by reducing administrative costs surely deserves a careful hearing. If the Russo bill is correct in asserting that hospitals' administrative and billing costs run to 18%, and that up to 45% of doctors' gross incomes can be spent on billing costs,[25] it may well be that simpler administrative procedures are the key to health care savings. In a recent editorial about proposals for health care reform, the *St. Louis Post-Dispatch* called the Russo bill the best of the lot.[26]

These comments on the Universal Health Care Act of 1991 conclude our survey of some of the major national proposals for reform of health care delivery in the U.S. Before moving to the next section, there are two points to be made about all the proposals we have considered. First, while the last two proposals call for national health insurance, none of the proposals calls for a national health *system,* i.e. a system in which the government owns enough hospitals and hires enough doctors to care for all Americans. In other words, every serious proposal made for health care reform in the United States recognizes the importance of retaining some aspects of the free market approach to health care delivery. Every proposal anticipates that patients would be free to choose which health plan or which doctors and which hospitals they want to supply their care. The proposals we reviewed became gradually more committed to government involvement in health care. There is room for debate about the merits of the different proposals. But none of the proposals wants the U.S. to move to socialized medicine, at least not in the strong sense in which socialized medicine would mean government ownership of the health system. On this point there seems to be a clear consensus.

Second, these proposals have talked in great detail about things which we should do in health care, things like providing universal access to health care, setting minimum health care benefits, cutting costs through simpler, more effective administrative procedures, etc. However, as I see it, none of these proposals explicitly raises the important question of whether there are some health care services we should not provide, whether there are some potentially beneficial health care technologies which we as a society cannot afford to develop, whether there are some classes of patients for whom the use of an existing technology would be inappropriate. Are there limits, in other words, in what we should be trying to do in delivering health care? Granting that some of the types of covert rationing which we cited earlier are unacceptable, might there be some morally reasonable types of health care rationing? Even if we admit the attractiveness of some of the reform proposals, will a suitable health care reform be possible in the U.S. if we do not consider the rationing or limits issue? Chapters 5 and 6 will look at this problem in more detail.

HEALTH CARE DELIVERY IN OTHER COUNTRIES

The last section outlined proposed changes in the U.S. health care system. Here we will take a brief look at health care systems in some other countries to see that programs of health care reform have been put into place elsewhere, with at least some success. Countries which have programs providing universal access to health care include France, Germany, Sweden, the Netherlands, Great Britain, Canada, and a number of others. While there are lessons which the U.S. can learn from all of these nations, we will focus on Great Britain and Canada.

Great Britain

Among the western nations, Great Britain was a major pioneer in moving toward a universal health system, with its first tentative steps in this direction having taken place early in the twentieth century. In the World War I years, the U.S. almost followed Britain's lead on health care delivery, and the whole history of health care in the U.S. might have been different had this happened. Later, in a radio broadcast to the English people in March 1943, Winston Churchill set out his hopes for a post-war England, and a National Health Service was one of his major priorities.[27] Churchill was voted out of office at the end of World War II, but in 1948 Great Britain did set up a true system of socialized medicine, i.e. a government owned health service.[28] Since this is the one thing which almost no one thinks the U.S. ought to do, it is quite ironic that a country to which the U.S. has been so close historically and philosophically has established a formal program of socialized medicine.

The British system has numerous shortcomings. There are serious complaints about certain medical services not being available and about other services taking a long time to get. There is concern that the British system impedes the development of new medical technologies. In public opinion polls, there is a somewhat smaller percentage of British citizens than Americans who think that they have personally been treated well by their health system (39% of British vs. 55% of U.S. citizens). It is true that there is a higher percentage of British citizens (27%) than Americans (10%) who think that their system as a whole is a good system, but neither of these figures is very encouraging.[29]

Great Britain has sought to diffuse some of the complaints about its health system by providing for the existence of private health services alongside the public system. These private services are well used. On the whole, the somewhat limited success of the British approach suggests that it may be just as well that the serious proposals for U.S. health care reform do not move in the direction of the British system. This is not to say that the British system is without merit; there is universal access to health care, and from an ethical viewpoint some difficult questions (such as the appropriateness of keeping someone alive for years or even decades in a persistent vegetative state) may be easier to address in the context of the British system than in the context of the current U.S. approach.

Canada

Because of the geographic proximity of the United States to Canada, and because some of the major health care reform proposals in the U.S. are similar to Canada's system, it is important for this book to consider the Canadian health care system which has now been in place for more than twenty years. The previous descriptions of the Physicians for a National Health Program Proposal and the Universal Health Act of 1991 (the Russo bill) have already set forth the essential structures of the Canadian system. Canada provides a national health insurance system administered through its provinces. But Canada does not set up a nationally owned system, in that physicians and health care facilities operate in the private sector. Once we understand this concept of public insurance coupled with the private delivery of health care, the main task is to make an assessment of the successes and problems of the Canadian system since it became fully operational at the beginning of the 1970s.[30]

First, and perhaps most important, the Canadian system provides access to a reasonably good level of health care to everyone in Canada. The exact specifics of which health care services are insured vary from province to province (e.g. only some of the provinces insure dental care), and there are debates about whether every single desirable medical service is provided. In general, however, the Canadian approach offers the same types of health services included in the major U.S. reform proposals, including hospitalization, doctors' services and a high level of public health measures. According to data assembled by Robert Blendon, about 60% of Canadians are very satisfied with the health care they have personally received (compared to 55% of people in the U.S.), and 56% of Canadians think their health care system as a whole is in good condition, while only 10% of Americans think that the U.S. system as a whole is in good condition.[31] While these figures suggest that the Canadian system has its limits, they show that Canadians are dramatically more satisfied with their system as a whole.

Second, Canada has been able to provide its universal access to health care with much greater cost efficiency when compared to the U.S. system. When Canada's current system went into effect in the early 1970s, Canada and the U.S. spent almost the exact same percent of their Gross National Products on health care (about 7%). Since then the percent of the Canadian GNP spent on health care has gone up slightly (to about 8.5–9%), but the percent of the U.S. GNP spent on health care has moved to the 12–13% range. A study based on the year 1985 showed that Canadians spent less for doctors, for hospitals, and for administrative costs. The most striking difference was in the area of administrative costs (billing, paperwork, etc.) where Canada spent only $21 per person, while Americans paid $95 each to cover the administrative costs of health care. On the whole, in 1985, the Canadian system cost $450 less per person, meaning that a similar system in the U.S. could have saved $100 billion dollars in 1985.[32]

If a Canadian-type system were put in place in the U.S., it remains to be seen exactly what would happen to health care costs here, but the reports on the financial savings of the Canadian system are certainly very important data. In themselves, the claims about savings made by some of the U.S. proposals (Kerrey, Russo, etc.) can sound like pie in the sky. The Canadian system offers some hard evidence to support these claims. Some critics argue that the faster growth of the Canadian GNP hides the fact that Canadian health care costs are rising at a rate similar to the U.S. rate of increase. But other studies point out that once the higher rate of Canadian inflation is considered, the difference in GNP growth between the U.S. and Canada is very small and the health care savings in Canada are very real.[33] To me this latter analysis seems more on target.

In reviewing all these positive accomplishments of the Canadian system, it is important to avoid simplistic thinking which suggests that Canada has solved all problems in health care delivery. In a very thoughtful critique, Canadian physician Dr. Adam Linton argues that Canada's global budgeting method may in the long run prove to be the most problematic aspect of the Canadian approach.[34] "Global budgeting" is the process whereby Canada's provinces set overall budgets for each hospital, but leave it to the hospitals to determine exactly how the budgeted monies received from the provinces will be spent. (Note that some of the U.S. proposals want to follow the same sort of process.) Dr. Linton argues that, in the early years of the global budget approach, Canadian hospitals were able to use their global budgets to be more efficient and to deliver a wide range of services at a reasonable cost. This is something similar to what happened in the U.S. when the DRG system first went into effect.

Nowadays, however, as more and more costly technological options become available, it becomes increasingly troubling for Canada to give controlled amounts of money to local hospitals and for the hospitals to have to figure out for themselves which technologies they ought to provide or not provide. Instead, Dr. Linton thinks that Canada will need to move toward some kind of public dialogue about what kind of health service it wants and does not want in an age of expanding technological options. He closes his article, as I closed my comments on the U.S. proposals, by saying that the rationing question will be the crucial question for the future of health care delivery.

Another interesting aspect of the Canadian system is the way in which it permits private medical insurance to be used. In Canada the substantial private insurance industry may only provide coverage for services which are not provided by the government system. These services can include things like special hospital accommodations, long term nursing care, and dental services (in some places). But there is no other insurance available for those services which the national insurance does cover, and thus there is no multiplicity of insurors covering the same services. If the U.S. adopts a single payer system, it will need to reflect on the place of supplemental private insurance.

A complete analysis of the moral value of the Canadian health care system must await the discussion of the theological/moral health care principles later in this book. But as a preliminary judgment, the Canadian system clearly feels like a breath of fresh air. The U.S. has much to learn from the Canadian experience. Canada's successes are not a complete answer, and ultimately the struggle for the just delivery of health care will challenge us to move beyond the Canadian system. But as of now, no other health care system in the world seems to be as just as the Canadian system.

RECENT LEGISLATION IN SOME U.S. STATES

In the last section we moved from proposed health care reforms to health care reforms which are already in place in some other countries. In terms of reforms which have actually begun to happen, we also need to note that recently there has been a trend toward health care reform legislation in a rapidly growing number of the U.S. states. It is doubtful that state action alone can solve the dilemma of just health care delivery in the U.S. Still, it will be useful to note what some of the states have been doing. It is not possible to review the new health legislation in every state, but we will look at recent developments in Hawaii, Massachusetts, New York, Minnesota, Maine, Vermont, and especially Oregon. As we look at these states, it will be clear that smaller states (such as Hawaii, Maine, Vermont, and Oregon) have found it easier to make major changes in health care than have the larger states whose health care systems are under even greater pressures.

Hawaii is the one U.S. state to have a program of universal health coverage in place and well established. Hawaii's program of universal access became law in the mid-1970s, and on the whole it must be considered a major success story.[35] There are several factors, however, which might make it difficult to export Hawaii's success to other states without a revised national approach to health care delivery. Hawaii's population is relatively small and its geographic circumstances are unique. Through the popularity of the Kaiser plan, etc., Hawaiians have had more than forty years of experience with health delivery systems which are not based on the fee-for-service model. Hawaii has a waiver from the federal law which forbids states from requiring employers with private health plans to participate in a state plan.

As an example of how it may be difficult to move Hawaii's success elsewhere, consider the state of Massachusetts which passed a law (originally set to go into effect in 1992) requiring employers to provide coverage for their employees or else pay an assessment to the state for health care. Because it requires an employer assessment, the law is under court challenge, and the effective date for the law has been deferred until 1995.[36] Anxious to avoid the legal difficulties of the Massachusetts approach, the New York State Health Department is proposing a program which retains existing health care payers such as employers but seeks to combine all these payers into a single payer system which will hopefully be more efficient. Recall, however, that in our review of the national proposals, we saw real doubts about the success potential of health reforms which retain too much of the present system.

Minnesota's new health care legislation imposes a 2% tax on hospitals, doctors, and other health care providers as a way of raising funds to enable Minnesota to supply health care coverage to the uninsured (with incomes of up to $37,000) whose income is high enough to render them ineligible for Medicaid.[37] It seems doubtful that such an approach could work as a basis for national health care reform. In the last chapter we spoke about the $17 billion in uncompensated care which doctors and hospitals are currently providing in the U.S. One wonders whether a tax on health care providers will simply force them to give up furnishing free care so that the end result turns out the same.

Some interesting health care reforms have taken place in the past few years in the state of Maine. Through the efforts of a coalition group called Consumers for Affordable Health Care, the state enacted the Maine Health Program, which, while not yet universal coverage, has made significant reductions in the number of uninsured by covering everyone under 100% of the federal poverty level. In response to the efforts of the same coalition, Maine became the first state in the nation to outlaw exclusions from health insurance solely because of pre-existing health conditions.[38]

In May 1992, Vermont governor Howard Dean (who is a physician) signed Vermont's new health reform law which aims to provide universal access to Vermonters by 1995. The Vermont law establishes a state Health Care Authority with three executives appointed by the governor. The authority will have the ability to bargain for the lowest cost for health care insurance for everyone in Vermont. The law enables the authority either to collect health premiums from individuals and groups or to establish a universal fund for health care to be supported through taxes. The governor favors the tax-based fund, making his approach very much like the Canadian single payer system.[39] What happens in Vermont in the next few years deserves to be observed very closely by the rest of the U.S.

While laws such as Vermont's are highly significant, the Oregon Basic Health Services Act of 1989 remains the most important of the recent state initiatives on the reform of health care. This law established the Oregon Health Services Commission, a group required to set priorities among the services to be provided to Medicaid patients in Oregon. Since Oregon's funding for Medicaid can only go so far, the commission's list of priorities means that lower priority needs will not be funded. What all this means is that Oregon has become the first U.S. state to use an explicit rationing approach to health care delivery.[40]

Besides establishing the Health Services Commission, the Oregon reform included a bill requiring all employers to establish play or pay programs by 1994, with these programs legally obligated to provide employees with at least the same level of benefits required by Oregon for Medicaid patients. The Oregon law also mandated the establishment of a state risk pool to provide coverage to the "uninsurable," i.e. those whom insurance companies will not cover. Fairly often, these two provisions are not described in popular commentaries on the Oregon plan, so that the impression is left that the Oregon plan is only concerned with Medicaid reform. When all the components of the Oregon plan are taken into account, the plan emerges as a more wholistic approach to health care reform.[41]

In reporting on the Oregon approach, the popular press highlighted the case of Coby Howard, a young boy who needed a bone marrow transplant for which state funding was not available. It was sometimes left unsaid that Coby Howard was not in remission and therefore not a good medical candidate for the bone marrow transplant.[42] But even granting the facts of this particular case and granting the other more wholistic elements which Oregon law is putting in place, it remains true that the Oregon approach clearly contemplates that some potentially beneficial treatments will not be made available to some persons.

There are some difficulties with the Oregon approach. To begin with, many find it troubling that the Oregon Health Services Commission's first emphasis is on the rationing of services to Medicaid patients, rather than to the population as a whole. In response, proponents of the Oregon plan argue that in the U.S. health care is already rationed to the poor in a fashion which is clearly unjust, so that the Oregon plan becomes a step forward. In addition, Oregon's proponents argue that the overall structure of the Oregon plan will ultimately lead to a similar delivery approach for all citizens, with insurance plans for the employed providing basic benefits but not every possible service.

Another criticism has to do with the way in which the Oregon commission has gone about setting its priorities. For example, if we take the perspective of the larger meaning of the human good, is cost effectiveness the best way to assess the meaning of the human good? The Oregon Commission is not unaware of this sort of criticism, and its 1991 priorities, while still open to debate, seem to be more sensitive to broader questions than were its 1990 priorities.[43]

Granting all of these questions, there is a crucially important basic insight at the core of the Oregon law: as a society with finite resources we cannot do everything which might offer some health care good to someone. In the future, all just systems of health care delivery may have to ask what we must supply and what we may choose, with regret, not to supply. Thus, whatever its limits, the Oregon plan bears serious watching and serious critique. The ethical aspects of the rationing question will continue to be with us as we move through this book.

In this chapter we have reviewed both potential and actual approaches to health care reform. We are now ready to move on to the second main part of this book, wherein we will engage in a process of theological and moral reflection on the major issues in the delivery of health care.

PART TWO

THEOLOGICAL AND MORAL REFLECTIONS ON HEALTH CARE JUSTICE

Chapter 3

THE HUMAN PERSON
AS MORTAL AND FINITE

In the next four chapters, this book will reflect upon the major religious and moral issues which, in my view, need to be brought to bear on today's debate about the just delivery of health care. This chapter will take up some basic questions of theological or religious anthropology, questions about who we are as human persons. The next chapter will address the specific ethics of care for the dying. Chapter 5 will address the meaning of human community, and Chapter 6 will focus on the theme of justice in relation to health care.

It will not be possible for this chapter to attempt an entire theological anthropology. There are, however, several themes from theological anthropology which are crucial to the ethics of care for the dying and thus to health care reform. These themes are death, sickness and suffering, asceticism, sin, the hope for resurrection, the value of life, creatureliness or finitude, and science in relation to human progress. We will consider these themes in some detail, especially as they relate to health care reform.

THE FACT OF OUR DEATH

As human beings, each one of us will have a very different history with a great variety of experiences. As we look toward our futures very little can be said with certainty about what will happen to each of us. In the final analysis, there is only one thing that can be said for certain about the future history of each of us, namely that one day each of us will die. Death thus becomes a basic fact of human existence, and every human person must work out some manner of integrating death into his or her approach to life. It is true that the human person has a spiritual nature, and that the Christian tradition believes both in the immortality of the human soul and in the resurrection of the human body. But the human spirit is by definition an embodied spirit so that death is inevitable for each of us.

Because death is such a basic reality in the story of human existence, our knowledge that one day we will die means much more to us than other universal knowledge that we all share as human persons. Knowing that we will die is not the same as knowing that the earth is round or knowing that water freezes at 32° Fahrenheit. Rather, our knowledge of our death is a part of our fundamental consciousness as human persons. Everything we do, say, or think is somehow marked by our awareness of death. Since so many of our values rest in our self-consciousness of death, it is very difficult to imagine what human life would be like if we knew that we were not going to die. The great theologian Karl Rahner tried to sum all this up by saying that death is present as an axiological (or value imparting) moment in every facet of human consciousness.[1] We live together on this planet as persons moving toward death. We live together here as persons peculiarly challenged to integrate death into our approach to life.

In saying these things about the central impact of death on human experience, I am in no way suggesting that we should like death or glorify death or develop some mystique which tries to pretend that the pain and loss associated with death are not real. It is true that death occurs in different contexts, so that we sometimes speak of it as timely or untimely. We can think, for instance, of our different feelings about the death of a person who dies after a long and happy life, about the death of a person who dies suddenly in the prime years of life, and about the death of a child whose whole life seemed to be ahead. But even granting these distinctions, death always outrages us and makes us feel that we are being punished (cf. Gen 3:22). We are saving the specific ethical questions about death for the next chapter. But here it must be clear that any sound vision of human life will support all reasonable efforts to prevent death. Our focus in this section is on the need for people to integrate death into their view of life, but this does not mean that death stops being death.

If we look more closely at the human challenge of facing up to death, it can be said that many aspects of modern culture go to great lengths to avoid this challenge.[2] As a result, large numbers of people in the modern world would rather not deal with death, but rather pretend that death never happens. Many examples of this psychology of death-avoidance could be cited. Here we will mention four such examples: athletics, advertising, the emphasis on sexuality, and the current interest in suicide and mercy killing.

In the area of athletics or fitness, it is surely true that exercise is a good thing, and that it can help maintain one's health. I do think, however, that some of the emphasis on physical fitness is related to a refusal to integrate the fact of death into the wholeness of life. Similarly, when we think about the enormous salaries paid to many professional athletes, it seems reasonable to ask just what values are behind such salaries. Is the rewarding of physical prowess at least partly the result of a worldview which would rather believe that death never happens, a worldview that glamorizes physical integrity beyond almost any other quality?

Similarly, while the advertising of products is an important part of our economic system, a great many contemporary advertisements seem to send the message that the product to be sold will make a person youthful, beautiful, physically strong, and sexually attractive. Many people in our society, especially young people, seem to get caught up in the naive worldview which advertisers and others often promote. The result is a consumer mentality in which people think that the purchase of more and more material goods will enable them to be in a constant state of happiness in a world in which death never happens. I am not suggesting that this worldview is present in all ads, but the consumerist, death-avoiding outlook on life is often very real.[3]

The links between sexuality and death are deep and fascinating. Both sexuality and death are related to the material side of human nature, for it is our materiality or embodiment which creates both the possibility of sexual pleasure and the fact of human death. A sound outlook on human life will acknowledge in a balanced fashion both the pleasure aspect and the death aspect of our humanity. If either sexuality or death is overemphasized, one's view of life becomes skewed. In the middle ages, there was at times a morbid, almost hopeless preoccupation with death, coupled with a good deal of repression of the meaning and goodness of human sexuality. Nowadays we seem to be in almost the opposite position. Sexuality is exalted as a topic of public interest (in entertainment, etc.), while the consciousness of death is often buried. Whatever side one took, the enormous interest in the Clarence Thomas hearings stands as an example of our society's emphasis on sexuality, to the exclusion of so much else including death.

Notable examples of our culture's desire to avoid dealing with death can be found in the growing interest in both suicide and mercy killing. In recent times we have seen *Final Exit*,[4] a book on suicide, move to the top of the best seller list, and we have seen a proposed law allowing mercy killing only narrowly defeated in the state of Washington. At first glance it might seem that an interest in suicide and mercy killing implies that people do want to face up to death and deal with it. Closer analysis, however, suggests that suicide and mercy killing are "easy way out" strategies, i.e. strategies which are aimed at helping people find overly simple ways to avoid dealing with the complexity of death. In saying this, I do not intend to judge the interior conscience of anyone who favors suicide or mercy killing. But I do think that Daniel Callahan is right when he argues that suicide and mercy killing stem from a desire to avoid facing up to death.[5]

The centrality of death as a fact of human experience and the need to face death honestly and realistically have obvious implications for the just delivery of health care. How can we know just what kind of health care we should be trying to deliver unless we have an adequate understanding of the place of death in human life? If we try to deny the reality of death, we are likely to make every conceivable attempt to prevent death, even when such efforts only serve to prolong dying and suffering. The result of such an approach will be ever greater health care costs, and more of the health care distribution problems we saw in Chapter 1. On the other hand, if we adopt the false assumption that we can make everyone's death easy, we run the risk of failing to provide life-sustaining treatments which people justly deserve, or even the risk of adopting mercy killing as a means of easy social management of health care delivery. Only with a sound human understanding of the meaning of death can we avoid these difficulties and have a suitable basis for a just system of health care delivery.

SICKNESS AND THE DILEMMA OF HUMAN SUFFERING

Just as we need a clear focus on the meaning of death, so too our approach to just health care calls for a suitable understanding of the true meaning of sickness and suffering as part of human life. In terms of a theology of sickness, recall the comments made earlier about death as a pervasive and ever present aspect of human consciousness and human value formation. It is true that the inevitability of death marks every experience in human life. It is also true that certain experiences or moments in human life raise a special challenge for us in terms of the death question. Certain times or focused moments make us especially aware of our death and of our need to integrate the fact of death into who we are. Numbers of such focused moments can be cited (including war, emigration, poverty, and divorce), but, without doubt, serious sickness focuses the human person's attention on death more than any other single human experience.[6]

At the time of serious sickness, a person's awareness of death causes the person to ask some very basic questions. What is life about? Is my life in good order? Am I in need of reconciliation with God or with my fellow human beings? Am I willing to accept my own death, once it becomes clear that it can no longer be prevented? Have I done everything I can to provide for the needs of my family and loved ones? If I am able to live for a while longer, are there any aspects of my lifestyle which I need to change? These kinds of questions make serious illness a very special time, a time for those around the sick person to have a special respect and reverence. In the end, sickness reminds us not only of the mortality of the human person; it reminds us as well of the dignity and worth of human life and human freedom. People in the middle ages were aware of all this when they first began to use the word "hospital," a word which referred in those days not so much to a place for curing as to a place where sick people could be welcomed with warmth, reverence, and hospitality.

Older Catholics will recall that before Vatican II the sacrament then called extreme unction seemed to focus on immediately impending death rather than on the reality of serious sickness which might over time lead to death. Happily, the restored Roman Catholic liturgy speaks of the sacrament of the anointing of the sick.[7] This changed title helps point out that sickness is a key human time, a time for prayer and human support. Many hospitals and nursing care facilities have developed fine programs of pastoral care so as to recognize these larger human dimensions of illness.

If the deeper existential implications of sickness are not recognized, sickness becomes little more than a mechanical failure to be repaired when repair is possible. Here again it should be obvious that reasonable efforts to cure sickness and to bring comfort to the sick should be praised and supported. However if health care planners and physicians are focused only on the physical repair of sickness, they may have a tendency to push for interventions in sickness which are clearly futile. They may fail to recognize that there comes a time to pause and pray, a time to stand back in respect and awe as the patient humanly faces her or his sickness. They may insist on using technologies whose ambience helps keep the patient from dealing with the deeper life issues which illness, especially terminal illness, can raise. We said at the beginning of the book that today's medical technologies can be truly wonderful. But only with an adequate philosophy and theology of sickness can we begin to form plans for the just and appropriate use of medical technologies for individuals and for society as a whole.

These remarks on sickness draw our attention to the even larger question of human suffering. Why is it that human beings suffer, whether through sickness, mental anguish, alienated relationships, poverty, or other tragic situations? For those who believe in God, why does God permit human suffering? For Christians, why did God himself suffer and die on the cross? People have struggled with these questions for centuries, and no one has ever produced a fully satisfactory answer. Certainly simplistic answers such as "suffering makes you into a better person" are to be avoided even though these answers contain elements of truth.

Among the modern theologians, Karl Rahner is especially helpful in addressing the suffering question. Rahner insists that our God is a radically holy and incomprehensible mystery, a mystery whose depths we will never fully exhaust, either in this life or in heaven.[8] From this perspective, the human acceptance of suffering becomes a significant faith event, an experience of trusting in the mysteriousness of the God whom we, like Job in the Old Testament, can never fully understand. It is with this awareness of the links between faith and suffering that the church focuses a major liturgical season (Lent) at least partly around the theme of suffering.

Clearly we can never glorify suffering. But if Rahner is right, suffering is ultimately a theological issue. If so, a meaningful social policy on death and sickness needs to come to terms with the deeper question of the place of suffering in human life. Facing this question will be very difficult, but the continuance of our present health care system may be even more difficult in terms of a Christian commitment to true justice.

ASCETICISM AND HEALTH CARE JUSTICE

The role of suffering in human life takes on another complex dimension if we stop to consider that across the centuries many religious traditions have encouraged a level of voluntary acceptance of suffering through various kinds of ascetical practices. Such ascetic practices are not limited to Christians; consider, for instance, the monastic communities which are part of some oriental religions. In the Roman Catholic context, members of religious orders take the vows of poverty, chastity, and obedience, and all Catholics are encouraged toward voluntary ascetical practices such as fasting and abstinence. In 1983 the Catholic bishops of the United States urged abstinence from meat on Fridays as a means for Catholics to commit themselves to the urgency of nuclear disarmament.[9] Such an approach shows that asceticism is not purely a personal matter. It touches our goals and priorities as a community.

When talking about asceticism we need to be careful not to glorify suffering so that we end up embracing some sort of spiritual masochism. But the widespread occurrence of ascetic practices suggests that many persons across history have realized that here on earth we do not have all the answers to life's problems. At times we need to stand back, voluntarily accept our limits, and trust in a gracious God who calls us to a higher destiny than we can work out on our own. For Christians, this higher destiny becomes explicit in the hope for resurrection and newness of life.[10] While non-Christians would not speak in these terms, their ascetic practices relate to similar value concerns.

To put this in another way, the ascetic tradition tells us that we need to grasp life lightly, that we sometimes need to be willing to let go of our own personal interests and priorities for the sake of higher values and for the sake of other people. Such a theology of letting go may be a crucial step in the movement toward health care reform.[11] If we accept the notion (as I think we must) that we do not have the ability to develop and apply every possible technology, then some hard decisions will need to be made about what to do and not do in terms of medical resources. If everyone who faces this question says "I want mine," the result will either be anarchy or access to health care based on power. It may be that only a recovery of the honorable ascetic tradition of past centuries and cultures will allow us to develop a sound health care system for the future.

SIN IN RELATION TO SICKNESS AND DEATH

In the last few sections, we have spoken about death, sickness, and suffering primarily as natural phenomena, as aspects of created human nature with which we must all come to terms. While it is true that death is essentially a natural reality, death also has important links with both human sinfulness and with our hope for final resurrection and union with God. Since these links can also help set the context for an approach to health care reform, we turn now to the questions of how sin and resurrection hope relate to death, sickness, and health care.

When we speak about sin and death, it is important not to make a formal causal link between sin and death, so that we end up saying something like: "So-and-so is dying because he or she is a sinner whom God is punishing." Such an attitude is not faithful to the notion of death as a natural phenomenon, and such an attitude seems likely to make us discriminate against giving care to certain dying persons whose lifestyle we may not like, persons such as criminals, drug addicts, and homosexuals. Especially in an era when society is addressing AIDS, such a linkage must be avoided.

However, even if we agree that death is a part of life, there are still two basic connections between sin and death. First, there is the fact that any person can die either as sinner or as saved. This means that as long as a person is living, she or he can choose to say an ultimate yes or an ultimate no to God.[12] She or he can choose to sin or choose to accept the gift of God's everlasting grace. From this perspective the time of one's dying is a critically important time of life. Earlier we mentioned the importance of praying for the dying, of standing by the dying with awe and reverence. Here we emphasize that a dying person is working out the core question of eternal salvation. All the more so this makes death a frightening prospect. All the more so this makes dying a time when people need love and care more than anything else, more than even the best medical technology. The link between sin and death in no way excuses us from providing truly necessary medical care, but the link does challenge us to be more aware of the true priority issues which confront someone who is dying.[13]

The second point of connection between sin and death flows from the traditional Christian teaching that human persons would not die, were it not for the original sin of Adam and Eve. Without getting into all the nuances surrounding original sin and its origins, the traditional Christian concept is that at the dawn of creation the human person was preternaturally gifted with immortality, i.e. spared from death. When sin entered the world, the human race lost the preternatural gift of immortality so that every human person must face death. Whatever else one might say, the traditional notion of death as the consequence of original sin suggests that death is a reminder of sin, that death and matters related to it can provoke all kinds of guilt and even tempt us to sin, e.g. to recommend treatments which a given patient does not truly need, to fail to tell a patient that he or she is dying. When we think about death, and about sickness and dying, we are very quickly brought into contact with the reality of human sinfulness.

This kind of link between sin and death suggests that the health care world, with its closeness to sickness and death, is very likely to be a world marked by sin. Sin can show itself in the health care world through a denial of death, through an excess individualism, through a refusal to bond with some of the dying, through an overly narrow emphasis on a scientific approach to health care, and in many other ways. Indeed, if we were to return to Chapter 1 and recall the problems in the current state of health care delivery, I think the conclusion would be inescapable that many of these problems are due to the sinfulness of the human condition.

In terms of a means of responding to the influence of human sin on health care delivery, it might be helpful to look at the traditional Catholic emphasis on frequent confession, even for persons who were not personally guilty of serious sin. Just why has the church emphasized the need for frequent confession? As I see it, frequent confession has been emphasized because of the church's insight that all of us need to live lives marked by a spirit of corporate repentance, whether or not we have personally committed sin.[14] In the health care context, I am not suggesting any specific rituals such as sacramental reconciliation, but I do think that our approach to just health care needs very much to be marked by a spirit of corporate repentance. If the health care context has strong links to sickness and death, and therefore to sin, a sense of repentance, of honesty about the problems of the past and present, would seem to be a key aspect of any move toward a more just system of health care.

THE HOPE FOR RESURRECTION

Surely the central vision-point of the entire Christian faith system is that all believers share in the hope for resurrection and new life beyond the grave. For believers, the resurrection of Jesus is not simply an historical event. Rather the faith-filled person believes that one day he or she will rise from the dead just as Jesus did. As St. Paul says, "If Christ be not risen from the dead, then vain is our preaching and vain too is your faith" (1 Cor 15:13).

This central resurrection faith would seem to influence the quest for just health care in two ways. First, the belief in human destiny beyond the grave becomes an ultimate statement of the dignity and worth of each and every human person. Because of our immortal destiny our rights as human persons stand out in bold relief. The outrage about the millions of uninsured persons in the U.S. fills our minds and hearts for many reasons. But for the believer, the status of all people as children of God hoping for resurrection becomes an eloquent summary statement of why we need a just health care system, of why each person has a claim on society for those health care services which are truly necessary.[15] We will have more to say about health care and human rights in Chapters 5 and 6, but the hope for resurrection is a crucial aspect of the human rights issues which pertain to health care.

Second, if the hope for resurrection reminds us that there is more to life than what we experience here on earth, then the power of the resurrection can make us more ready to face up to the fact of death, more ready to accept the fact that the time for death may have come. Care is needed in how this is said. The hope for resurrection does not make death stop being death. It does not take away the pain of death or absolve us from any reasonable efforts to prevent death. But if it is true that many in our society are unduly afraid of death, and if it is true that medicine is sometimes tempted to overtreat even when death is inevitable, it may be that the hope for resurrection will give us a better focus on the meaning of death, a focus which will be good not only for dying individuals, but for society as a whole as it seeks to provide health care more justly.

Of the issues we have just addressed (death, sickness, suffering, sin, and resurrection), it is the resurrection theme which is most clearly and explicitly Christian. Thus the resurrection theme helps raise an important question. Since we are stressing here so many traditional Christian concepts, are we implying that one must share in Christian faith in order to develop a truly just health care system? My point in writing this book is to reflect theologically on our health care system, so it is both natural and necessary for me to raise theological questions which relate to health care. I would not claim, however, that only theists, Christians, or Catholics can work out a just health care system.

What I would say instead is this: In the past few sections we have been looking at some ultimate questions about the meaning of death and life. While someone who is not a Christian would not answer these questions in Christian terms and symbols, I do not think anyone can move toward just health care without asking and answering the foundational questions which are being asked in this chapter. Moreover, I think that anyone who wishes to move toward a more just health care system will need to answer these questions with a sense of the openness of life, a sense that there is more to life than the concrete physical needs and desires of concrete individuals. If one's sense of life focuses only on the individual and only on the here and now, it could well be that the move to just health care will be an impossibly daunting task, a task which will get hopelessly bogged down in the demands of a rugged individualism. No, I do not expect atheists and persons from other traditions to become Christians. But anyone who wants just health care must be willing to ask the foundational questions about who we are together on this planet.

The Marxist philosopher Ernst Bloch rejected theism, but he did say that human persons needed to have a sense of a "Messianic Frontal Space" out ahead of them.[16] Bloch's frontal space is an example of the open view of life which any person must have in order to face the issue of just health care.

THE MEANING AND VALUE OF HUMAN LIFE

So far in this chapter, we have looked at issues related to the meaning of death and sickness. Our reflections would be very incomplete, however, if we did not also examine the meaning and worth of human life, especially human life on the biological level. How could we know our just obligations to preserve life and health without first coming to terms with the meaning of life?

To begin we must acknowledge that human life has a sacredness or sanctity about it. The Roman Catholic tradition has often referred to the sacredness of human life, especially by referring to life as a gift over which we human persons do not have an absolute dominion.[17] The bishops of Vatican II stressed the sacredness of human life and mentioned a number of unspeakable crimes against life which must always be avoided.[18] In a secular context, the U.S. Declaration of Independence alludes to the sacredness of human life by using the famous phrase "the right to life." From very early in human history, it has been popular to say that the greatest sin is murder, because murder takes a human life. Without doubt, therefore, life makes a very primal claim on human consciousness. This is why health care and its delivery is such a pressing moral issue. We are not dealing with just any human value. We are dealing with life. This also is why in the end it seems more reasonable to think of medicine, nursing, and other types of health care work as vocations. Medicine, nursing, etc., are clearly professions, but as ministries to human life, they are even more clearly vocations.

In today's world, the mention of the theme of life's sacredness makes it hard not to think about abortion and about the Roman Catholic Church's long-standing tradition on the inviolability of fetal life. The church's clear opposition to euthanasia also comes quickly to mind. While I agree strongly with the church's stress on the sacredness of fetal life and with its opposition to euthanasia, it is not my purpose here to articulate the theology and ethics of either abortion or euthanasia. Instead, my purpose is more general: to emphasize the sacredness of all of human life, to stress right to life as it applies to every human person.[19] It is precisely because of such a wholistic life-centered ethic that the question of just health care delivery rises with such force or impact on us. How can we talk about the sacredness of human life without being concerned about the availability of health care services which can sustain and enrich human life?

Once we say that human life is a sacred value, we need to move on and ask exactly what kind of value human life is. Is life a value simply in and of itself? Or is life a value because it serves as the foundation for other values? Because of the sacredness of life, this is a very delicate question. It cannot be answered casually. The fear is that if we say life is a value because it exists for other values, we may appear to be undercutting the sacredness of life. Any answer which does suggest that human life exists for other values will need to be developed with great care and precision.

But in the final analysis it seems more compatible with Catholic vision and with sound philosophy to say that human life is an instrumental value, a value which ultimately exists so as to serve other values. St. Thomas Aquinas wrote that the final end of the human person is happiness with God in heaven.[20] More recently, Pope Pius XII wrote that life, health, and all temporal activities are in fact subordinated to spiritual ends.[21] The gospel of John evokes this same context when it defines eternal life as the knowing of God (Jn 17:3). Similarly we can argue that life is sacred at least partly because it gives us the opportunity to form relationships with other people and to build up the dignity and worth of the human community.

It is not possible here to probe all the ethical nuances behind the comments of St. Thomas or Pius XII, and it is clear that they would never permit their statements on the meaning of life to be used as grounds for abortion or euthanasia. Nor would the theme that life is subordinated to spiritual ends in any way deny that life is a crucially important value, a value which always deserves respect, a value which makes all other human goods possible. But it remains clear that the traditional Catholic thinking about the subordination of life to spiritual ends has helped generate the Catholic position that we do not need to do everything possible to prolong the life of a dying person. In the context of the present book, this thinking about the prolongation of life can have a very important impact on the quest for a just health care system.

Once we begin to think about human life's role in support of other values, we can begin to see some of the rationale behind some other major ethical dilemmas which have beset humankind across history. In earlier centuries people took long and perilous journeys across the oceans, even though they knew they might lose their lives instead of finding the better world for which they hoped. People have volunteered for risky medical experiments, even though they knew that life could be lost in the process. A common consensus continues to exist holding that war can sometimes be justified. As a theologian I was struck that, while some wondered whether the specific war against Saddam Hussein was just, and while others called for a careful reformulation of the just war theory in light of modern weaponry, relatively few thinkers in the debate about the war against Iraq questioned the underlying concept that war can sometimes be justified.[22]

In stating these examples, I am not attempting to develop a fully precise analysis of all the ethical thinking which undergirds them. Such an analysis would call for the explanation of the difference between direct and indirect attacks on life, the difference between proportionate and disproportionate attacks on life, the difference between innocent and guilty human life, and many other factors.[23] My point here is simpler: to show that life is a value which exists in relation to other values. With such an awareness, it is not difficult to defend the classic Catholic notion that we need not take every conceivable step to prolong life.

When we speak about life being sacred and also speak about life being subordinated to spiritual ends, it is hard not to reflect on the contemporary debate which pits the sanctity of life against the quality of life. In many ways I find this to be an unfortunate debate, and I believe that Roman Catholic theology embraces solid themes found on both sides of the debate while at the same time rejecting the extremes which sometimes crop up on both sides of the debate.

Drawing upon the sanctity tradition, Catholicism accepts the crucial insight that we may never directly attack innocent human life. This is the basis for the church's opposition to abortion and euthanasia. But when some persons use the sanctity of life as a basis for arguing that we must always prolong physical life, the church's awareness that human life is subordinated to spiritual ends leads to a different conclusion. Many proponents of the sanctity of life position will agree with the church on this issue. Those who do agree with the church reject the vitalism which marks the thinking of some who would call themselves proponents of the sanctity of life.

In accord with the quality of life side of the debate, the church has long accepted the insight that we are not required to prolong a burdensome physical life for someone whose death is at hand. The

U.S. bishops' Pro-Life Committee has recently reaffirmed this and other related insights drawn from a "quality of life" perspective. However, the bishops' focused and limited acceptance of such insights does not mean that they are adopting a formal quality of life stance[24] or accepting many of the other positions which are sometimes advanced as "quality of life" arguments. In general there are three ways in which the Catholic outlook differs from the position of some quality of life proponents.

First, Catholicism would never accept arguments which would interpret our obligations to prolong human life in terms of social convenience, e.g. arguments which might suggest that we could refuse life-saving treatments to a retarded child simply because the child's family finds care for the child to be socially burdensome. Second, Catholic teaching holds that a person's very serious medical condition (and therefore poor life quality) can only be used as a ground for non-treatment in cases where the burden arising from the treatment is clearly excessive when compared to the benefit to be gained, with this situation most likely to be found in the lives of persons who are in a terminal condition. Third, Catholic theology recognizes that sometimes we will be unsure as to whether other value issues such as the achievement of justice can truly be compared with the value of physical life. In these cases, Catholic theology (unlike some "quality" advocates) tends to hold that we must give the benefit of the doubt to physical life and act in its favor. Before the Persian Gulf war, for example, most Catholic leaders in the U.S. argued against the war because they were not sure that the arguments for the justice of the war were clear enough to outweigh the arguments in favor of human life.

In summary it can be argued that the Catholic position opts for a very careful selection of insights from the sanctity of life and quality of life perspectives. In my view such a balanced position constitutes the most sensible approach to the debate about the quality and sanctity of life.

There is one way in which the sanctity/quality debate is important in the context of health care justice. The sanctity perspective helps make us aware of those health care services which we ought to provide to every human being while the quality perspective can help us be aware of life-prolonging measures which we might reasonably choose not to provide in a future health care system. In the end, decisions about what to provide and what not to provide will be critically important aspects of a reformed health care system.

HUMAN FINITUDE AND ECOLOGY

Many of the issues we have looked at in this chapter remind us that we are finite, that we are creatures and that God is our creator. The awareness of our status as finite creatures brings a certain humility into our lives, a certain awareness that the world is God's world rather than ours. In much modern thought, including medical thought, there is a tendency to think that we humans are in complete charge of the world, to think that the world is mere raw material which we can play with in any way we wish. Medically such a "we are in charge here" viewpoint can lead to a totally uncritical development of medical technologies, a development which gives little consideration to the impact that medical technologies can have on the social and the natural worlds. The naive overconfidence in our ability to conquer death and the tendency to portray health care professionals as the high priests of modern times both stem from this overconfidence in human potential and human power. We need therefore a dose of humility, a willingness to praise God who is in fact our creator and the Lord of the universe.[25] We ourselves are stewards rather than the lords of creation.

Of course there is a legitimate realm of medical research and progress. But sound theology has always held that our life on this planet is both a problem to be solved and a mystery to be contemplated. If we forget that we are creatures, life becomes too exclusively a problem to be solved. In my view, a good deal of the difficulty with health care today comes from a forgetfulness of the mysteriousness and contemplative nature of human existence.[26] This problem is by no means limited to health care professionals, nor is it fair to say that all health care professionals are unmindful of their status as creatures. But the issue is there, and it is hard not to think that a better health care system might emerge from a more honest recognition of our status as creatures rather than creators.

Among moral theologians, the great Protestant scholar James Gustafson has most eloquently argued for the need to move away from the anthropocentrism which has dominated so much western thought in recent times. In his classic work *Ethics in a Theocentric Context*, Gustafson brilliantly retrieves the notion that this is God's world rather than our own.[27] Perhaps more than any other contemporary Protestant scholar, Gustafson is thoroughly familiar with and quite approving of Roman Catholic thought. He does feel, however, that Thomas Aquinas' confidence in human learning may have been pushed too far by some moderns, and that we all need to be reminded by the great reformers that we and our world are under God's judgment. Hence, Gustafson articulates his "preference for the Reformed Tradition."[28] Even if one does not accept all of Gustafson's presuppositions, he articulates a refreshing challenge to today's world, a challenge with much potential as a foundation for working out a human and humble system of health care reform.

A number of themes might be used to exemplify the notion of a world which belongs to God rather than to us. One of the most important such themes is the question of ecology. More and more we are aware of the problems which human interventions are creating for plants and animals, for soil and air. Beyond the specific threat of ruined forests and extinct animal species lies the even greater concern of gradual global warming with its long term potential for destroying much of the earth's life as we now know it.[29] We will treat Pope John Paul II's social teaching at greater length in Chapter 5, but one of the most significant things about the holy father's social teaching is that he has become the first pope to call the world to account in the area of ecology. He does this most formally in his great encyclical *Sollicitudo Rei Socialis*.[30]

The ecology question has some important parallels to the health care delivery question, so that what we learn about ecology can help shape our approach to health care delivery and vice versa. Here we shall cite three examples of ways in which an ecological consciousness can give shape or focus to our efforts to deliver health care more justly.

First of all, since ecology makes us aware that the physical world around us is at risk, it certainly be argued that ecological risks should be an important factor for medicine as it seeks to assess its own priorities. If it is not possible for medicine to develop every single feasible medical technology, a good case can be made for not developing those technologies which are more likely to damage the environment. Care is of course needed in making such decisions. A technology with a high potential benefit may have a relatively low ecological risk and thus be deserving of development. The question of animal rights also comes to the fore in this same context. While I would not agree with those who would rule out all use of animals in medical research, concern for animals can add an important ecological caution to the development and delivery systems of modern medicine. For instance, if there are other reasonable ways of developing a given technology besides animal research, such ways are to be preferred.[31] If only one of two equally valuable medical technologies can be developed, the one less dependent on animal research is to be preferred.

Second, the ecological crisis has taught us all a greater sense of reverence for the world around us and for the harmony of its natural processes. Earlier, when speaking about sickness, I emphasized that sickness is a time which calls for a sense of respect, prayerfulness, and hospitality in the presence of the sick person, whether or not we are able to cure the sickness. I think that the ecologist's reverence for nature and the health care community's reverence for the sick have some notable similarities in terms of basic attitudes. Surely, reverence for the sick and dying is even more important than reverence for nature, but the two reverences can help support one another.

Third, the ecological movement has helped restore to humanity a true sense of limitation, a realism which holds that the world is not made of infinitely manipulable raw material. Thus there are some things which we cannot do in the name of progress, even if we would like to. In other words, ecology has helped us recover the earlier traditions of asceticism, of grasping life lightly. We saw earlier that medicine needs to be marked by a sense of limits and asceticism, and it may well be that ecology can teach medicine some important lessons in this area. None of this of course exonerates medicine from offering patients truly necessary care. But there is a certain spirituality of ecology which may in time become a helpful aspect of the spirituality of health care delivery.

SCIENCE AND HUMAN PROGRESS

In the context of all we have been saying about human finitude and human limits, there is one more task that remains in our reflection on theological issues which can help ground a more just system of health care delivery. This last issue is a theological evaluation of the scientific method which has been so pivotally important in the development of modern health care services. Near the very beginning of this book I spoke about the wonders which modern medicine has wrought through science, so there is no justification for any attack on medical science as such. Despite occasional tensions, a positive attitude toward science has marked Roman Catholic theology ever since the thirteenth century when St. Thomas espoused Greek natural law philosophy with its high faith in human science and learning. Even with such a positive outlook, however, there is room for some critique of the place of science in medicine, for a critique which might help medicine move

toward a more just system of delivery. In what follows, we shall offer
three points of critique.

First, the very nature of scientific knowledge is that it tends to be
divided into a wide variety of categories. Such a pluralism of sciences
is essential for the growth of scientific knowledge, but it also creates a
world in which each scientist has a rather narrow view of the world, a
world in which each scientist can be said to know more and more
about less and less. Karl Rahner points out that every act of scientific
learning is like an act of renunciation, in that the scientist deliberately
excludes from view certain types of information in order to focus in
detail on the information which she or he wishes to discover or expand.[32] Because of this narrow focus (perhaps well exemplified by an
instrument such as the microscope) science can tend to ignore larger
questions about the meaning of life, and the diverse specialties of
different sciences can make it hard for scientists to communicate with
one another. The larger more wholistic view of life can be missing.

Of course this larger view is not absent in all serious scientific scholars. Many of them are fully aware of the deeper human questions.
Many of them have developed interests in the liberal arts such as literature, music, painting, and dance, i.e. on aspects of human life and learning which focus us on a sense of wholeness and ultimately on a sense of
God. Nonetheless, it remains true that science as a method can tend to
ignore larger questions about the meaning of human life. It goes almost
without saying that modern medicine has many roots (both positive and
negative) in the scientific outlook on life. For medicine to come to terms
with the crisis in health care delivery today, it seems that medicine will
need to recover, at least in part, its traditional status as an art.[33]

Second, besides its tendency to a narrow focus, science has a
strong impetus toward expansion and progress, toward the production of results. If science is not moving out to new frontiers, it has a
sense of failure. For many in science, it is almost unthinkable that a
given scientific breakthrough not be implemented, once the technological expertise has been developed to put the breakthrough into
place. Some of the researchers who were working on recombinant
DNA felt that their work should be completely unrestricted by public
policy, even though there were some uncertainties about the kinds of
new and potentially dangerous organisms which might be developed
through recombinant DNA. In this chapter I have several times
praised the work of Karl Rahner, but in one of his articles even
Rahner seems overly convinced that science ought to do everything
which it is possible for it to do.[34]

As a science, medicine can often share in this almost unrestricted

sense of making progress through ever new and expanding technological developments. But should medical technologies always be developed and put into use? Are we wise enough, for instance, to decide
justly which children should receive liver transplants? Or are there
times when medicine needs to pause and reflect more on whether or
how to use given technologies? Such questions come from a larger
than scientific perspective, and they may be a crucial part of health
care reform.

Third, science has about it an intensity, a pace or speed in which
movement seems more or less constant. Because there are so many
frontiers, and because science wants to conquer them all, science
never wants to stop moving. As such, science makes little connection
with the contemplative dimension of life, little connection with the
sense of wonder and ecstasy which marked the thought of the great
rabbi Abraham Joshua Heschel and so many other thinkers.[35] This of
course does not deny that numbers of scientists, as human persons,
have developed a very genuine contemplative spirit.

The modern hospital very often reflects this high speed, high
intensity view of life. Often there is so much to be done by the hospital
staff that there is little time to stop and think about what is really
happening. Without doubt, top speed and top intensity are needed in
many medical situations, but life, health, sickness and death are about
more than speed and intensity; they are also about waiting, watching,
and hoping, and ultimately about trusting in God. None of this means
that health care should abandon its roots in modern science. But, to be
fully human, health care must be more than science.

In summary, this chapter has tried to present a theological anthropology for health care, i.e. a summary of human dispositions, attitudes, and sentiments which seem crucial for the achievement of
health care justice. Surely other similar issues could have been considered, but hopefully the key themes of a theological anthropology for
health care are clear. As the chapter ends, the reader may have two
questions. First, would a revitalization of the dispositions, attitudes,
and sentiments about life and death which we have just reviewed be
sufficient by itself to bring about the reform of health care? Definitely
not, for there are questions of economics, politics, justice, and morality which must also be considered. Second, will any reform of health
care be possible unless we revitalize the dispositions and sentiments
described in this chapter? Again, definitely not. My judgment is that,
without the religious foundations just described, our society will never
be able to face up to the many other issues which need to be part of
overall health care reform.

Chapter 4

THE SPECIFIC ETHICS OF CARE FOR THE DYING

The last chapter surveyed basic theological attitudes about life, death, sickness, and dying. Besides these basic attitudes, theology, especially Roman Catholic theology, has developed a very clear set of ethical principles to be used in making concrete decisions about the care of individual patients. As I see it, a careful understanding and implementation of these ethical principles has the potential of accomplishing a great deal to ameliorate the present crisis in the delivery of health care. Thus, the goal of this chapter will be to present an overview of the fundamental ethical principles which pertain to care for the dying. To help make these principles clear, some concrete case issues will be discussed. But in the discussion of these difficult concrete cases it will not be possible to offer a complete analysis of all the pertinent issues.

Organizationally, the chapter will be divided into five sections. First, there will be a summary statement of the Catholic principles on care for the dying. Second, we will enhance our understanding of the principles by looking at several typical cases to which they apply. Third, we will study the process by which individual death and dying decisions are made. Fourth, we will see how the Catholic principles apply to current controversies such as medical futility and active euthanasia. Fifth, we will see what impact the Catholic principles can have on the problem of the just delivery of health care to all people, or, to put it in another way, we will seek to enlarge the Catholic principles on death and dying from a personal to a social context.

CATHOLIC PRINCIPLES ON DEATH AND DYING: A SUMMARY

The Importance of Caring

Much in this section about principles on death and dying will focus on things which we may not need to do for dying patients. Thus it helps to begin by pointing out the one thing we must always do for dying patients: give them care. Part of the very nature of our humanity is that we are bonded to one another in such a way that we owe one another certain basic loyalties or obligations. While a number of such loyalties could be cited, it should be crystal-clear that one of the most basic loyalties we owe to one another is the loyalty of watching, waiting, keeping company, standing by, and giving care to one another as we go toward our deaths. Whatever else we need to do or not do for specific patients, the obligation to be there giving care always remains. It is an obligation or covenantal commitment which falls to the entire human family, but it rests in a special manner on health care professionals. It is also an obligation which is foundational to the whole notion of human rights in health care. Many contemporary authors have helped to articulate this call to keep company with the dying, but in my view the work of the late Paul Ramsey was especially helpful on this point.[1]

Members of the modern generation might not be aware that the well-known cartoonist Garry Trudeau has a great-grandfather who was a very famous figure in the history of health care in the United States. In the 1870s, Dr. Edward Livingston Trudeau was brought to the village of Saranac Lake in New York's Adirondack Mountains. At the time of his arrival Dr. Trudeau was so sick from tuberculosis that he only expected to live for a few months, and he hoped that the cool mountain air might make his dying days more comfortable. But Dr. Trudeau lived for more than forty years, founded the great TB sanitarium at Saranac Lake, and spent his entire life working on TB and caring for patients with the disease.[2] His son and grandson became doctors and followed in his footsteps. Much of the early work on TB is quite significant today because TB patients often faced prejudices similar to those faced in our times by AIDS patients.

After Dr. Trudeau's death, the great American sculptor Gutzon Borglum executed a beautiful statue of Dr. Trudeau reclining in one of the famous Adirondack chairs with a lap robe pulled up over him. On the reverse of the statue, Borglum carved in French the words of the motto which seemed to summarize Trudeau's whole career at Saranac Lake. The words are *Guerir Quelquefois, Soulager Souvent, Consoler Toujours* ("Sometimes to cure, often to relieve, always to bring consolation"). I have always felt that these words are a perfect summary of fundamental health care ethics. We cure when we can, relieve pain when we can, but we are always there keeping company, bringing care and consolation to the dying.

The Basic Catholic Tradition:
Ordinary vs. Extraordinary Means

The precious obligation to care for the dying carries with it the implication that we cannot always cure people, that death will happen to all of us in the end. Thus we need a set of principles to help us decide what we must do and not do for dying patients. In the Christian era, this matter first received significant attention in the sixteenth century. In 1536 the Catholic theologian Francisco Vittorio discussed the question of whether a person always needed to use food to preserve life. Toward the end of the century, Domingo Soto wrote about the question of whether a religious superior could compel a religious community member to prolong his or her life under the vow of religious obedience. Finally, in 1595 another theologian, Domingo Banez, articulated the famous distinction between ordinary and extraordinary means of preserving life and health. This distinction was further developed in the next century by Cardinal De Lugo.[3]

According to the ordinary/extraordinary distinction, all persons are called upon to take ordinary steps or measures to preserve their life and health, but no one is obligated to use extraordinary means to preserve his or her life and health. I believe that Roman Catholic moral theology deserves real credit because it developed this distinction several centuries before anyone else in modern society gave serious consideration to the matter of what we must do and not do for the dying.

If we look at the ordinary/extraordinary distinction as it existed from its inception until the mid-1950s when so much in medicine began to change, the most striking note about the distinction was its tone of common sense realism.[4] It was said, for instance, that whenever a medical intervention brought a patient excessive pain, the intervention was extraordinary. Likewise, if a medical intervention caused a patient grave inconvenience, such an intervention could be considered extraordinary. This meant that there was no obligation to take steps such as moving to another part of the country for the sake of one's health. It was also said that whenever a medical intervention was very expensive, it could be considered extraordinary. By this criterion, a great deal of what is offered by the modern health care system could be considered extraordinary. Even if we were to accept some greater costs as ordinary today, it is hard not to think that the common sense outlook of many of the earlier proponents of the ordinary/extraordinary distinction would see many of today's medical technologies as extraordinary and beyond what is required. We of course must argue out of the context of the

1990s, but there is much to learn from the simplicity of earlier views on the ordinary/extraordinary distinction.

Another significant fact about the earlier writings on this matter is that many of the earlier authors were not as focused on an isolated interpretation of the term "means" as we might think when we hear the term "ordinary means." Instead, a number of earlier authors knew that the means had to be related to the person before a judgment about ordinariness or extraordinariness could be made. Writing in the 1950s, the well-known Jesuit moralist Gerald Kelly discusses two examples from the work of Cardinal De Lugo which help to clarify the point about the means relating to the circumstances of the person. Today the examples strike us as quaint and whimsical, but they make an important point.[5]

The first example concerns a person who has a close friend who is being burned at the stake by his enemies. The person has enough water to slow down the fire which is killing his friend, but not enough water to stop the fire and save his friend's life. In this case De Lugo held that the water, even though it is the ordinary way to put out fires, need not be used. The second case has to do with someone who is being unjustly starved to death. His friends might be able to bring him a little food, but not nearly enough to prevent his eventual death by starvation. Need the person slow down his inevitable death by eating the food? Again De Lugo said no, even though we would ordinarily use food to prevent starvation.

A fuller analysis would be necessary in order to show all the implications of De Lugo's examples for today's debates. But even without such an analysis, the examples help us see the wholistic nature of the ordinary/extraordinary tradition. This tradition considers not only the nature of the means but the effect of the means on the person. In the next section we will review the modern description of ordinary means as those which offer reasonable benefit in comparison with the burdens they impose. This description has clear roots in the works of Kelly and De Lugo.

The Ordinary/Extraordinary Distinction Today:
Efforts at Reformulation

Because modern medicine can do so many phenomenal things, a number of today's medical technologies can be argued to be quite ordinary from a medical perspective which often looks at technologies apart from the person. For this reason, some authors have sought to reformulate the ordinary/extraordinary distinction in a fashion that more faithfully captures the common sense, person-oriented character which the distinction has possessed since its inception in the sixteenth century. Richard A. McCormick has argued that the key element is whether or not a given technology offers a specific patient a reasonable hope of benefit.[6] Very significantly, the Congregation for the Doctrine of the Faith, in its famous 1980 *Declaration on Euthanasia,* suggests that the classic ordinary/extraordinary distinction may be less clear today, and that some may prefer to speak of proportionate and disproportionate means.[7] The text goes on to say that doctors may sometimes judge that in certain medical circumstances the investment in technologies and personnel is disproportionate to the results to be expected. Doctors may also judge that in some cases the technologies to be used will impose on the patient a level of suffering out of proportion with the benefits which might be gained. This sort of language with its emphasis on proportionality by no means abandons traditional Catholic thinking on care for the dying. But this language clearly implies that we are speaking of means in relation to persons instead of means in the abstract. Echoing formulations used by many others, the Maryland Catholic Conference recently spoke about the "benefits and burdens of the treatment to the patient." Such language does not focus on an isolated evaluation of the treatment, but on the human impact of the treatment on the person. I think such a formulation helps show the true Catholic sense of the distinction between ordinary and extraordinary means.[8]

Contrasts with Other Views

To help explain the Catholic "proportionate means" view of death and dying, it might help to contrast the Catholic approach with several other viewpoints. The Catholic "proportionate means" view very obviously contrasts with the vitalists who say that absolutely everything must be done to preserve life with no other considerations having any place at all. The Catholic view also is in clear contrast with those who see medical choices as a matter of pure personal autonomy, so that there is always an absolute right to demand or to refuse treatment. The Catholic view insists that life decisions are to be made on the basis of principle rather than personal whim. This point about solid principles will be very important when we consider whether society can set any standards about what it is obligated to do for people in the area of health care.

The Catholic view is also distinct from any views which argue that death and dying decisions are purely medical in character. Catholicism is concerned for the whole person, and not just with the person's body. Similarly, the Catholic view is distinct from those who would base death and dying decisions on issues related to the convenience of society. Catholicism has too much of a sense of the dignity of the individual human person to accept arguments based on social convenience. For a more thorough exploration of all of these contrasts, the work of Richard Sparks, C.S.P. is especially helpful.[9]

In describing these contrasts with other views, I have refrained from describing the position of those who insist that, for a technology to be non-obligatory, the heavy burden must be in the technology itself rather than in technology's relationship to the overall condition of the patient. In this view, even if the patient's condition is greatly burdensome, simple technologies must always be used, even if these technologies only prolong the patient's suffering and dying. As we have seen, the Catholic tradition does expect us to use technologies which bring people care and comfort, even as they die. However, as we saw in the earlier manualists' examples, the Catholic tradition does not look at the means alone, but rather at the efficacy of the means in relation to the circumstances of the sick person. Thus, it is within the scope of the Catholic tradition to argue that a technology which only serves to prolong great burden for the patient (for instance the burden of a painful death) need not be used even if it is a simple technology.

The view which focuses on the simplicity or the burden of the means is the closest of all the contrasting views to the Catholic view. Indeed there are times when the focus on the means will be a clearer criterion than the circumstances of the person, so that prudence will call us to make the character of the means the decisive moral factor. Especially when we get into the area of social policy, it may be very important to attend to the greater clarity which sometimes can be found by examining the character of medical technologies in and of themselves.

SOME TYPICAL CASES

The main focus of this chapter is to describe the Catholic moral tradition on death and dying, so that we can see what impact this tradition might have on our ways of approaching health care justice. Thus it is not necessary for us to go into a detailed analysis of how the Catholic tradition applies to specific cases. I do think, however, that an understanding of the Catholic approach to some of the specific cases is critically important for a wholistic grasp of the Catholic ethic of care for the dying. With an understanding of some typical cases, we will be much better able to become attuned to the social justice implications of the Catholic tradition on care for the dying. In what follows we will consider how the Catholic tradition might approach five concrete cases.

Emergency CPR

The first case area has to do with the use of emergency cardiopulmonary resuscitation (CPR), i.e. with reviving a person who has suffered a cardiac arrest. Often such an attempt at revival is called coding a patient, because so many hospitals have some sort of code system by which they summon a response team to try to revive a patient who has suffered a cardiac arrest. Without doubt, medicine has made enormous progress in the use of emergency CPR over the past twenty-five years. There are many patients who can be brought back from the very edge of death through the use of emergency CPR.

At the same time, however, it must be acknowledged that CPR can be an invasive technology with the compression of the chest and other means that are used. Surely when a person's health status is unknown, or when it seems very likely that a person may recover substantially from the cardiac incident, the use of CPR is indicated. But what about the patient who is clearly in the process of dying anyway? Are we obligated to use CPR if the only plausible result is that the patient will suffer along for a few more days, hours, or weeks? Most experts in ethics would say that we are not required to use CPR is such cases, that its use does not offer the patient a reasonable hope of benefit.[10] Studies have shown that of patients beyond a certain age and in certain medical categories, only a very tiny percentage who are successfully coded will not die during their current hospitalization.[11] No-code decisions can therefore clearly be beneficial for some patients. In addition such decisions, while they should not be made on larger social grounds, can have important implications for the conservation of health care resources.

A clear process ought to exist in all health care situations for stipulating whether or not someone is to be a code or a no-code patient. If a no-code decision has been made on solid grounds, the transfer of the patient to a hospital (from the patient's home or from a nursing care facility) is not of itself a reason to reverse a previous no-code decision. Similarly, if it is decided that a medical procedure such as radiation or surgery could bring care and comfort to an already hospitalized no-code patient, the procedure should not constitute grounds for automatically suspending a previous no-code decision.[12]

Pain Management

In some situations, a patient who is dying is dealing with a significant amount of pain and in need of relief from the pain. While pain-killing medications can help to keep dying patients comfortable, their usage can contribute to the breakdown of the human system, meaning that the time of death will be hastened. This is especially true if gradually increasing amounts of medication are needed to control the pain. The classic Catholic principle of the double effect would not seem to rule out the use of even gradually increasing levels of pain medication in such situations. The fact that the time of death may be hastened is the indirect result of a medical procedure undertaken for a good purpose, i.e. the relief of pain. Granted that in these cases death is usually imminent anyway, there seems to be a proportionate reason for permitting the death to occur a bit earlier.

Two cautions are needed on this matter. First, we are not speaking here about the use of a massive amount of pain medication all at once with the specific intention of ending a person's life then and there. Second, decisions about pain management need to be made from a wholistic and spiritual sense of the person, not on physical grounds alone. For instance, a given dying patient may have an important personal/spiritual agenda for which she or he needs a higher quality of consciousness, even if this consciousness involves a good deal of pain.[13] Perhaps such a patient needs to deal with a long lost son or daughter who is finally reappearing as the patient is dying. The use of enough pain medication to severely limit the consciousness of this patient would be inappropriate, even though such a use of pain medication might be appropriate for another patient in similar circumstances. The *Declaration on Euthanasia* to which we referred earlier has some helpful and important guidance about pain and consciousness.[14]

Dying Patients and Second Diseases

Another famous dilemma in the ethics of care for the dying occurs when a person who is dying of one disease gets a second disease which is easily curable. The means for curing the second disease are simple or "ordinary," but all that the cure of the second disease accomplishes is the prolongation of the first disease. Is the curing of the second disease morally required in this circumstance? Is the curing of the second disease for the proportionate good of the patient?

Pneumonia is probably the most typical example of this sort of case. Fairly often in the end stages of cancer and other terminal diseases, a person will get pneumonia. What sort of obligation is there to treat the pneumonia? First, it should be noted that some aspects of pneumonia treatment such as suctioning will serve to bring comfort to the dying patient. Since we must always care for a patient, such comfort-bringing measures would be required. But what about the vigorous treatment of an imminently dying patient's pneumonia with antibiotics? If we look at the patient as a whole person and not as a set of discrete symptoms, I think the case can be made that a cure of the pneumonia is not for the proportionate good of the patient. Hence, something like vigorous antibiotic treatments may not be required.[15]

A Multiplicity of Diseases

Fairly often in medicine it can happen that a dying patient has a number of different things wrong with him or her. No one of the patient's medical difficulties can be said to be clearly leading to the patient's death. However, when all of his or her symptoms are taken together, the clear conclusion is that the patient is dying. Sometimes it can be difficult to assess such cases because several different physicians may be involved in the patient's care, with no one physician having a clear picture of the patient's prognosis. In any event, once such a case is assessed, and it is clear that the patient is in fact dying, can it be moral to terminate some of the elaborate treatment modalities which have been undertaken in behalf of the patient?

This kind of case can surface in various ways. Perhaps such a patient is on kidney dialysis. Perhaps the patient's breathing is being assisted by a ventilator. Whatever the measures are, in the face of the onset of death, it can be reasonable to discontinue them since they no longer offer the patient a reasonable benefit and thus are no longer proportionate to the patient's needs. Shortly we will speak about how such decisions get made and about the implications of such decisions on the availability of health care resources. But for now the point is that such decisions can be for the patient's good.

Artificial Nutrition and Hydration

Of all the specific case areas, the question of whether we must always supply patients with artificial nutrition and hydration support (intravenous needles, nasogastric tubes, gastrostomies) is the single most delicate question. We will review this question here, but without getting into all the issues of theological debate which relate to the nutrition/hydration issue.

Since we must always care, and since nutrition and hydration are so closely related to the call to care, it is clear that in the great majority of health care situations we are required to provide nutrition and hydration. For Catholics and other Christians who have a strong faith in the eucharist, the judgment about the importance of nutrition and hydration becomes even clearer due to our faith that Jesus is specially present to us in the elements of food and fluid. Therefore the discussion of artificial nutrition/hydration begins with the assumption that we should provide nutrition and hydration support. Arguments to the contrary should only be made with great care, and it is particularly important that we not try to solve this issue on any grounds of social convenience.

To say, however, that we normally assume we will provide nutrition and hydration does not necessarily prove that we must do so in every conceivable case. In 1984 the U.S. Bishops' Committee for Pro-Life Activity spoke about the presumption in favor of providing nutrition and hydration to dying patients.[16] Presumptions state what we plan to do and what we ordinarily do, but the fact remains that presumptions can sometimes be set aside, in the face of overriding evidence to the contrary. For instance, if a patient's digestive system has failed so completely that he or she cannot digest any injected fluid as nourishment or hydration, and if attempts to nourish without using the person's digestive tract are also not possible, then there is no reason to attempt nutrition/hydration support since it simply cannot be done. In this case, attempts at nutrition and hydration support are not proportionate to the patient's circumstances. Similarly, if a patient is very close to death, and it is clear that, in the short time which is left, the lack of artificial nutrition/hydration will not cause any lack of comfort, the dignity of the person's dying hours or days might suggest the appropriateness of removing or not starting the artificial nutrition/hydration supports.[17] Such a course is fairly often used with cancer patients as death approaches. Such patients may be conscious and still able to take some food and water orally which is fine.

By far the hardest nutrition/hydration case has to do with the patient who is in the persistent vegetative state (PVS). This dilemma is particularly acute because, while the patient will never recover consciousness, the patient will probably not die if nutrition and hydration are continued. The patient might live for years or even decades in the PVS. Great care must be taken in determining whether or not a patient is actually in a PVS. There are well-established neurological criteria which must be followed in assessing the PVS, and a time period of one to three months or more is necessary to make the judgment.[18] But in the end there are PVS patients and the need to make a sober judgment about what we owe them.

If we go back to some of our earlier discussion about the meaning of life and about ordinary and extraordinary means, it seems to me that the moral question is whether artificial nutrition/hydration is proportionate or appropriate for the PVS patient. To put it another way, the question is about the burdens and benefits of the treatment (artificial nutrition/hydration) for the patient. Does the treatment bring more burden than benefit, or vice versa? Surely physical life is extended, but is there more benefit than burden for the person as a human being?

A review of the medical-moral literature of the past decade shows that the more common opinion is that artificial nutrition/hydration is not proportionate for the PVS patient, that the burdens of this treatment are such that its benefit is not a reasonable benefit. From this perspective, artificial nutrition/hydration supports are not morally obligatory for the PVS patient. Among the many authors who hold this opinion, the Jesuits Richard McCormick and John Paris are perhaps the best known.[19] Personally I am in agreement with the viewpoint that artificial nutrition/hydration is not required for the PVS patient, chiefly because I think this viewpoint is more in accord with the Catholic tradition on the prolongation of life, as this tradition has developed since the sixteenth century.

Those who hold the opposing view argue that being alive in a persistent vegetative state is of sufficient benefit to the patient that the artificial nutrition/hydration supports are morally required. The statement prepared as a working paper for the Pope John XXIII Center (by William E. May and others) is probably the best known summary of the arguments for the obligation to provide artificial nutrition/hydration to PVS patients, but there are also noteworthy statements of this position by the late John Connery and by Gilbert Meilander.[20]

Like theologians, individual bishops and bishops' conferences show a division of opinion on the obligation of supplying artificial nutrition/hydration to PVS patients. Some individual bishops and some state bishops' conferences (such as Texas and Washington) have issued statements which are rather open to the idea that artificial nutrition/hydration may not be obligatory in some of these cases. Other bishops and state bishops' conferences (notably Pennsylvania) have argued that the supplying of artificial nutrition/hydration to PVS patients is a clear moral requirement. But interestingly the Pennsylvania bishops do not absolutely rule out the possibility that a case might occur in which the burdens of the artificial nutrition for a PVS patient are such that it would not be required.[21]

On April 2, 1992, the U.S. Bishops' Pro-Life Committee issued a statement on this matter which holds that the removal of artificial nutrition/hydration supports should not be deemed appropriate or automatically indicated for the entire class of PVS patients. This means that the moral presumption in favor of nutrition/hydration remains in place for PVS patients. The Pro-Life Committee's statement acknowledges the division of theological opinion on the issue. It recognizes that not all the pertinent questions have been addressed by church authority, and it concludes by describing itself as the committee's first word, and not their last word on this difficult issue.[22]

One underlying question connected with the nutrition/hydration discussion is whether a terminal condition is always required before we can withdraw any of today's elaborate medical technologies from a given patient. Clearly, a terminal diagnosis helps give any judgment about the non-use of technology the sharp patient-centered focus which Catholic teaching requires. But might there be other factors besides terminality which give a case the clear patient-centered focus which is necessary for the judgment to withdraw or not to initiate a given medical technology? Great care must be taken, but my judgment is that other sufficiently clear factors can exist, especially if the patient has expressed his or her own wishes on the issue at hand.

Another underlying question has to do with the relation of the nutrition/hydration discussion to the issue of active euthanasia. Sometimes those who oppose the withdrawal of nutrition/hydration from the PVS patient seem to take their position at least partly out of fear that the opposite position will lead to euthanasia. We will consider the whole question of euthanasia further near the end of this chapter, but in general my view is that we should have confidence in the persuasive character of the church's anti-active euthanasia stance. With this confidence, we can strive for sound and correct judgments on PVS cases in and of themselves, without worrying that these judgments will erode the church's teaching on euthanasia, even if the judgments do permit the withdrawal of nutrition/hydration from PVS patients.

I mentioned earlier that there is a majority opinion on PVS patients and artificial nutrition/hydration among theologians and health care ethicists. But the debate about this issue will not be resolved quickly. In the end what may be most interesting is that increasingly both sides in the debate are using philosophical categories such as proportionality or burden vs. benefit of the treatment for the person as they articulate their views. I think that this kind of language, regardless of the conclusions on specific cases, helpfully avoids both uncritical emphasis on the social burden of caring for a PVS patient and a focus on technical functioning of the treatment as disconnected from the human good of the patient. With this kind of framework, my hope is that we can move toward a more responsible and more socially just approach to the delivery of health care, even if we do not fully resolve every difficult case.

These comments on nutrition/hydration conclude our summary of some of the specific areas to which the Catholic proportionate care tradition applies. At the end of the chapter, we shall look back at some of these cases to see what they mean in terms of possible routes to health care reform.

HOW DO THESE DECISIONS GET MADE?

In this section we are going to look into the process for making decisions on matters such as codes, pain management, etc. We shall consider both the standard account of health care decision making and an important Catholic critique of the standard account. As we shall see, the Catholic critique is by no means a rejection of the standard account, but it does bring some important additional perspectives to bear on the process of health care decision making, perspectives which might help in the quest for social justice.

In the standard account, the first priority in health care decision making is what the patient herself or himself wishes. This priority comes from a sense of the inherent dignity and freedom of the patient. Often, in the kinds of cases we have reviewed, the patient will be able to say what he or she wants. This can be the case in code/no-code decisions, pain management decisions, withdrawal of technologies such as dialysis, etc. If the patient is able to express his or her views, health care providers are normally responsible for following those views.[23]

When the patient cannot speak for herself or himself, the natural and normal thing is for the patient's family to speak for the patient. Catholic teaching recognizes this,[24] and in many of the states in the U.S. there are substituted consent laws which explicitly recognize the right of family members to make health care decisions for a person who is incompetent, i.e. unable to speak for herself or himself. Usually such substituted consent laws establish an order of priority among various family members so that the doctors will know to which family members they are most required to pay attention. It should be noted that a family's right to direct the care of a patient is not absolutely unlimited. If parents want to refuse life saving treatment for their child, the courts will often take the decision making power away from them. In 1990 the U.S. Supreme Court ruled that a state might legitimately request clear and convincing evidence of the patient's wishes before nutrition//hydration are withdrawn from a PVS patient.[25] The wishes of the family may not constitute the clear and convincing evidence of what the patient himself or herself wanted. So there are limits on family decision making, but the normal presumption is that families can speak for incompetent sick persons.

But what about those cases in which a patient has outlived all other members of his or her family? Such cases are not rare in these times when medical technology enables substantial numbers of patients to live to very old ages. Also, what about those patients whose family systems are so broken down and divided that the family cannot express its views in any coherent fashion? Who speaks for these patients when they become incompetent?

In almost every state there are two major legal options for patients who cannot count on their families or who have no families to speak for them. These options, known by the general term *advance directives,* are the *living will* and the *durable power of attorney for health care.* The living will is a set of written directions for a patient's health care once the patient becomes terminal. These directions bind both the caregivers and the patient's family. With a durable power of attorney for health care, a specific person is appointed to speak for the patient, and the directions given by the person with the power of attorney are legally binding. Many people execute both of these advance directives, which is perfectly acceptable. From the point of view of Catholic theology there is nothing formally wrong with either approach.[26] The durable power of attorney does provide the advantage that the person speaking for the patient can not only know the patient's wishes but also talk to the doctors and find out the actual diagnosis, prognosis, and treatment options. To me at least, this seems a little more human than a mere set of written directions.

The living will and the durable power of attorney must be executed in proper legal form, but both forms are quite easy to execute. In addition it should be noted that if a patient has expressed his or her health care wishes to his or her doctor, and if the doctor has documented these wishes in the patient's medical records, such documented medical records can also stand as legally binding evidence of what should be done for an incompetent patient.

The primary purpose of advance directives is to foster the human rights of individual persons as they make health care decisions. It is interesting to note, however, that advance directives will often be used in a manner which leads to a careful stewardship of health care resources, i.e. persons will use these directives to rule out costly non-beneficial treatments. The end result may well be that the growing interest in advance directives will contribute to the development of a more just health care system by avoiding overtreatment and by making more resources available for use by those who are presently uninsured. It would be wrong to force advance directives on people as a means of achieving a more just approach to health care. But to the extent that the wise use of advance directives moves us toward greater health care justice, all well and good.

Earlier I said that there was both a standard account of advance decision making and a Catholic critique of the standard account. The Catholic critique can perhaps be focused by looking at some of the educational efforts and publicity about the Patient Self-Determination Act, a recent federal law which requires all hospitals, nursing homes, and all other facilities receiving Medicare or Medicaid funding to ask all patients whether they have executed any advance directives concerning their health care. Much of this publicity tends to portray a patient's health care decisions as matters of purely arbitrary choice, so that the patient is completely free to choose whatever he or she wants or does not want.[27] Some of this emphasis on the freedom of the patient's choice ties in strongly with the undercurrents of individualism which mark so much of American life. The context is not a context of what I ought to do, or of what responsibilities I may have toward my family or toward society in my health care decision making. Rather the context is that what I want to choose is right simply because I want to choose it.

It is at this point that the Catholic critique arises. Catholicism agrees with the dignity and freedom of the human person, and with the necessity of the person's making basic health care decisions. Catholicism insists, however, that a patient's health care decisions must be based on a sound assessment of the medical facts and even more so on a solid set of moral principles. From such a perspective, patients are not free to request or refuse anything and everything. Rather they are free to request or to refuse only when their requests or refusals are grounded in the understanding of proportionate care which we described earlier. The *Declaration on Euthanasia* makes it clear that to assess proportionality the patient or those speaking for the patient must enter into dialogue with the doctor about just what a given treatment will accomplish or not accomplish.[28] All of this implies that there are some important community standards at stake in terms of what medical care is required or not required.

This Catholic critique of excess individualism in health care decision making is important and helpful. But the critique should not be taken as questioning the dignity and worth of the human person. Nor does the critique deny that in many cases the best medical course of action will be unclear, meaning that patient choice, like any choice in conscience, remains a crucial factor in health care decision making. What is always necessary is for patient choice to be based on sound commonly shared principles about the meaning of life and death. Later on we will explore the impact of these commonly shared principles on health care reform.

TWO CURRENT ISSUES:
MEDICAL FUTILITY AND ACTIVE EUTHANASIA

Medical Futility

We can add to our understanding of the ethics of care for the dying and of the implications of these ethics for social justice by looking at two significant current debates concerning the role and mission of health care. The first of these debates concerns the question of medical futility. Often in this chapter we have spoken about the burdens and benefits associated with some medical treatments. We have argued that there may be cases in which careful reflection determines that the burden of a treatment is such that its use is not morally required, even if the treatment does offer some benefit. Perhaps in these cases it might be argued that a treatment is not required because it is relatively useless or relatively futile. But what about those cases in which the lack of medical benefit is so overridingly clear that the level of futility might be said to be absolute or at least approaching absoluteness? It is this latter more absolute notion of medical futility which has become an important theme in the debate about stewardship of resources and the just delivery of health care.

In recent years medical futility has been much discussed in the journal literature on medicine and ethics.[29] The major point of the discussion is this: Can we continue to construe all decisions related to life-extending technologies as matters of pure patient choice, so that the patient (if insured or otherwise able to pay) is always guaranteed of getting whatever he or she wants in terms of life-extending tech-nologies? Or might it be that the use of some medical technologies for certain classes of dying patients is so clearly contraindicated medically that health care providers are not obligated to provide these technolo-gies, even if patients ask for them?

History is an important factor to consider in looking at this ques-tion. In an earlier cultural context (e.g. before the mid-1960s or there-abouts), it was clearly assumed that doctors could make decisions on what to offer based on the notion of medical appropriateness. Even today, apart from the context of certain types of life-extending treat-ments, the assumption remains that a doctor or hospital can refuse to provide a treatment which simply is not germane to the patient's care. If the patient persists in asking for such a treatment, the doctor can withdraw from the case.

On certain types of life-extending issues, however, the assump-tion is different. Without regard for the standards of good medicine and without any legal requirement, a patient is thought to be free to ask for whatever he or she wants with the understanding that the doctor and health care facility must provide it. For example, in the case of emergency CPR, it is assumed that the patient must be resusci-tated unless he or she requests otherwise. This is so in spite of the fact that, in a certain set of medical cases, it is becoming increasingly clear that the very high probability is that the patient may never recover consciousness, may suffer greatly, and may live for only a very short time. More work needs to be done to sharpen our under-standing of this type of code case, but the point is that for some patients the use of CPR is medically contraindicated because a pro-portionate result is not to be expected from its use. Do the hospital and the doctor have a moral right to refuse to provide such treat-ment? Would any grounds other than a complete vitalism justify a moral requirement that such a treatment be provided? While the answer to these questions must focus on the good of the patient, the social implications of such questions should be obvious in a country which desperately needs to find ways of being more efficient in the delivery of health care.

Before we try to answer the futility question, an important cau-tion is in order. We need to be very careful in terms of just how we go about defining futility. In the current literature, several different de-scriptions of futility have surfaced. Some of the current definitions of futility seem to have the clear understanding of disproportionate means which we find in the Vatican's *Declaration on Euthanasia*. But other current definitions of futility sound more like social inconvenience or like something the doctor would rather not do, but without any hard criteria to verify the proposed treatment's virtual total lack of effectiveness. If we are going to consider an affirmative answer to the futility question, such an answer should apply only to the cases where clear and defensible criteria are present, i.e. those cases in which there is a clear public consensus that the level of futility is approaching the absolute.[30]

If one sees patient autonomy as the ultimate moral value, there is no ground for ever refusing a treatment which the patient requests. However, if one sees patient autonomy as a value grounded in deeper moral values such as a shared set of common principles about the meaning of life and the meaning of health care, then it might be possible, in limited cases, to refuse to provide medical treatments which are clearly futile. Precisely because Roman Catholicism does see human life in terms of a common set of moral principles, there would seem to be a basis in the Roman Catholic view of life for refusing to provide clearly futile medical treatment. I offer this conclusion with the awareness that more needs to be done to develop an adequate notion of medical futility.

A tougher related question is whether, for the sake of some higher good, a society might ever have grounds to choose not to provide medical treatments which are not manifestly futile, but which have only a limited benefit. Before answering this question, we will need to reflect on the traditional understanding of the common good, a project which will be taken up in Chapter 6.

Active Euthanasia

In speaking about active euthanasia or the direct termination of another person's life, I want to mention two main themes, the arguments against euthanasia, and the roots of the interest in euthanasia in our own times. On the first theme, nothing which I have said in this chapter about the non-obligatory character of some medical technologies in some situations should in any way be understood as a legitimation of active euthanasia which is a very different moral reality. In the context of active euthanasia it helps to recall Paul Ramsey's argument that even apart from the rights of the individual patient, active euthanasia would be very disruptive of the social fabric of society, and especially disruptive of the character of the relationships between health care providers and patients. What would life be like in the health care world if patients construed providers as the persons who would ultimately do them in? This problem might be focused differently if euthanasia were performed by persons other than providers, but the moral problem would still remain.

Recently Daniel Callahan has written against euthanasia and repeated many of Ramsey's same arguments against it. Callahan has appealed to reports from the Netherlands (where euthanasia is allowed in some circumstances) which seem to show that Ramsey's concerns of a generation ago may be coming true in the Netherlands. The law in the Netherlands is carefully limited, but besides the legal cases of euthanasia, there are substantial numbers of euthanasia cases occurring in the Netherlands in violation of the law. Another of Callahan's concerns is that many pro-euthanasia arguments come from an overemphasis on self-determination, i.e. from a rejection of the classic Catholic notion that our dominion over our life is not unlimited. All this helps to show the need for the Catholic corrective on self-determination which I mentioned earlier. John Paris has also published a very helpful critique of the arguments for active euthanasia.[31]

The clarity of the moral arguments against euthanasia do not mean that the debate over euthanasia will go away any time soon. For a long part of 1991, it looked as though the initiative legalizing euthanasia in the state of Washington might have been passed by the voters. Only a determined effort by organizations of health care providers, by religious leaders and by others helped prevent the initiative from passing, but the tension about the issue is likely to continue.[32] As I mentioned earlier, it is not my purpose to judge the sincerity and possible good faith of some of the persons who favor active euthanasia. But from the point of view of both moral standards and social policy, the Catholic position against euthanasia remains clear and compelling.

The concern about the growing interest in active euthanasia has led some persons to be very fearful of implementing the traditional Catholic ethic with its position that we need not use extraordinary or disproportionate means to keep a person alive. These persons worry that the use of the traditional Catholic ethic will place us on a slippery slope toward euthanasia. I grant the concern about euthanasia, but I disagree with the fear of the traditional Catholic position. One of the oldest principles in ethics is *abusus non tollit usus,* i.e. that potential abuses ought not take away legitimate uses of a set of principles. Besides, we shall see that there is an important argument which shows that the sound use of the Catholic position may actually lessen the drive toward euthanasia and in the process increase the prospects for a more just health care delivery system.

In terms of the roots of the interest in euthanasia today, I earlier cited Daniel Callahan's point that for many euthanasia is a sign of an unwillingness to address the fact of death in a realistic and human manner.[33] I think Callahan is much on target about this point. There is also another critically significant factor in today's debate about euthanasia: the fear so many people have that they will be over-treated when death approaches. This fear leads them to favor eutha-nasia as a way of protecting themselves against overtreatment. This book began by focusing on undertreatment, on the millions of per-sons who are either uninsured or underinsured. But in the high-tech world of modern medicine, overtreatment is very often a problem as well. The rhetoric of "do everything possible" can easily prevail with-out a consideration of the deeper human good of the patient. In my experience of many years of service as an ethical consultant in hospi-tals, I have frequently dealt with overtreatment issues, so I under-stand the fear.

It is in this context that the brilliance of the traditional Roman Catholic view begins to shine very brightly for me. If all patients could be sure that they would be treated with the common sense realism of the Catholic view, I think many of them might be a lot less fearful of things like overtreatment and painful death. This might very well leave patients much less inclined to push for active euthanasia.[34] Espe-cially today, when modern medicine does have the means to keep the great majority of dying patients comfortable and the ability to give the real care which Dr. Trudeau found so central, it seems that a medical world is possible in which the drive toward active euthanasia might be lessened. I say this in full awareness of the difficulty involved in suffer-ing and dying, but, as the last chapter mentioned, death is a part of life which we must face in a human way.

I am concerned that if we spend a great deal of energy in the years ahead debating the pros and cons of euthanasia, it may be all the harder to work toward health care reform, since the energy for such reform might be sapped by the euthanasia debate.[35] Thus, if the traditional Catholic ethic, with its sound arguments against overtreat-ment, can become more widely accepted, this ethic may help take some of the power out of the euthanasia debate. In the process, the traditional Catholic ethic might serve to provide a better context for the discussion of health care reform.

THE CATHOLIC ETHIC OF CARE FOR THE DYING
AND THE POTENTIAL FOR HEALTH CARE REFORM

The Catholic ethic which we have now reviewed is moving and worthwhile in and of itself. But what about the impact of this ethic on the quest for a more just health care system? As I see it, the Catholic ethic (which is held in similar forms by many other reflective persons) can have three favorable implications for the achievement of a more just approach to health care delivery.

First, the Catholic ethic has the potential for significantly reducing the problem of overtreatment of patients. We just alluded to the overtreatment theme when speaking about euthanasia, but this theme's import is very great in the context of health care justice. I have had a number of opportunities to speak with hospital financial officers about the annual operating losses which their institutions sometimes experience. Very often it seems that, if a hospital has lost five million dollars for its operations in a given year, a very substantial part of that loss can be attributed to the management of ten or twelve patients in whose cases it can be fairly asked whether the treatments given were for the patients' good, either medically or morally. Hospital structures such as quality assurance and utilization review have helped to reduce overtreatment, but the fact is that many overtreatment cases remain. If most or all of these overtreatment cases could be eliminated, major sums of money could be saved. This could both reduce the cost of health care and make more funds available to care for the uninsured and the underinsured.

A great watchfulness needs to mark the way in which we speak about this matter. The priority remains that we must make good decisions on behalf of each patient in terms of what treatment is truly for the patient's good. Any campaign to get persons to execute advance directives simply to save hospitals money would be wrong. Similarly, ethicists usually argue that those who make the decisions on the care of an individual patient should be separated from any health care managers whose primary job is to worry about costs. Such steps would help to assure that costs alone never serve as the basis for refusing proper care.[36] The point to be made then is this: If we use a sound ethical basis for deciding what is proportionate to the human needs of each patient, such proportionate decisions, when reviewed in an aggregate fashion, will have a substantial favorable effect on the cost of health care. To say this in another way, the proportionate decisions which stem from the Catholic ethics of care for the dying will be an exercise of good communal stewardship. This will be so, even granting that some individual health care decisions will of necessity remain quite costly.

Some readers might want to ask at this juncture whether I think that better observance of the Catholic ethic on patient care will alone be sufficient to reform our health care system. I do not. I think that it will also be necessary to reassess the overall purposes of health care vis-à-vis education, housing, economic growth, and other social concerns. But I do think that elimination of overtreatment and the implementation of something like the Catholic ethic is a sine qua non for health care reform. If we do not succeed in dealing appropriately with the overtreatment issue, we will not find the road to health care reform.

The second potential contribution of the Catholic ethic of care for the dying to the debate on health care delivery stems from Catholicism's rejection of a one-sided notion of autonomy and from Catholicism's insistence that individual health care decisions need to be based on sound moral principles which can be held in common by society. We saw this rejection of all-out autonomy and the insistence on common principles in the Catholic approaches to advance directives and medical futility. If it is true that elimination of overtreatment, important as it is, will not suffice to reform health care, then we very much need a national dialogue to restore some common assumptions about who we are as a people and about what goals we can share together, not only in health care but in life as a whole. Our next two chapters will explore this question of U.S. community in great detail. For now the point is simply that the Catholic approach to dying drives us toward the principled approach which will be essential if we are going to move to a common social dialogue.

Third, I believe that the Catholic approach, with its clear vision of how to care for the dying, can help us avoid certain distractions or side-roads which might otherwise cause us to travel long detours instead of facing up to the issues which are crucial for health care reform. We have already seen the grounds for the Catholic conviction that euthanasia, in addition to being morally wrong, is not a suitable means to health care reform. Similarly, Catholicism would insist that science and technology alone cannot solve the health care delivery problem since we will always be faced with the question of whether and how to use our medical technologies. Also, the Catholic ethic will help us reject any pure social utilitarianism which tries to solve the health care delivery issue by ignoring the dignity and worth of each individual person. These and other related examples show the potential of the Catholic ethic for keeping us focused on what is really important in health care delivery.

Surely there are some tensions and difficulties in the Catholic approach to care for the dying. The moral thinking about the nutrition/hydration issue is not completely clear. There is the important unresolved tension between those who lean more to the efficacy of a medical means in itself and those who lean more to the impact of the means on the person as a whole. So it would be wrong to naively state that the Catholic view is fully developed on all health care issues. Thus the Catholic tradition can learn from other thinkers and other religious traditions. But the fact remains that the Catholic ethic of care for the dying uses its solid principles to arrive at a wonderful common sense of realism about life, death, and suffering. For this reason the Catholic ethic offers much to the debate about health care reform.

Chapter 5

BUILDING COMMUNITY: THEOLOGICAL AND PHILOSOPHICAL ROOTS

The preceding two chapters have shown us much about the meaning and ethics of health care for the individual person. However, concern for the individual person is not enough, especially in our culture where concern for the individual can so easily turn into an isolated individualism. To move toward meaningful reform of health care we need an awareness of who we are for one another, an awareness of what sort of community we are called to be here on earth. Only from such a sense of communal responsibility will we have a context from which to make specific health care reforms. As I mentioned earlier, Chapters 5 and 6 will use an organizational pattern similar to the pattern of Chapters 3 and 4. This chapter will establish some basic theological/philosophical understandings of community, and then the next chapter will discuss some of the ethical norms for community building and health care which stem from the theology and philosophy of community.

If I were writing this book thirty years ago or more, I would have almost certainly dealt with only philosophical issues related to community building. Before Vatican II, Catholic authors hardly ever discussed the theological roots of our political and social community here on earth.[1] Happily, since the council there is much more awareness of theological anthropology in all of its communal implications. Theological anthropology tells us that the life of faith of the human person as a child of God summons the person to a strong social responsibility for other human beings and for the structures necessary to support human community. In the first half of this chapter I will summarize three themes which help to ground the communal demands of a Catholic theological anthropology: the meaning of God as Trinity, the meaning of Christ and the church, and the meaning of the human person as a lover of his or her neighbor. Because these themes will not be developed to the extent of many other issues in this book, their treatment will have a different tone than many of the issues which were discussed earlier. But even though the treatment will be brief, I think it is crucial for persons of faith to see that they must approach an issue such as health reform out of communal faith experience and not simply on philosophical moral grounds.

But the advent of theological anthropology does not mean that the Catholic philosophical grounds for community have lost their importance. Thus the second half of the chapter will discuss three concerns coming from a philosophical anthropology, i.e. from the more traditional Catholic approach to the place of the person in the community. The three philosophical concerns to be considered will be the natural possibility of building the human good through structured community, the role of civil law in generating community, and the need for a disciplined life of virtue and character. Overall, this combination of theological and philosophical themes means that the chapter will review six community building themes. In each of the six, we will try to tease out some significance for health care reform.

THE TRIUNE GOD AS SOURCE OF COMMUNITY AND AS MYSTERY WHICH GROUNDS OUR HOPE

Often we think of God as being over and above us, as being very distant from our concerns and problems. In this context we are unlikely to think that the core character of our faith in God might in itself be the ground for a move to health care reform. However, the central and unique Christian notion about God—the idea that God is a Trinity of persons—has a great deal to say about the kind of care which we owe to one another in all areas of life. We need therefore to examine our faith in the Trinity in order to try to grasp it a little more deeply and see what implications it may have for the project of this book.

For many Christians, faith in the Trinity is like an abstract piece of theological baggage which we have stored in some sort of religious attic but which comes in for relatively little consideration in terms of the practical living of daily life. In trying to take the Trinity out of our religious attic and dust it off a bit, there is no denying that the Trinity is a profound mystery which none of us will ever fully grasp or understand. Nonetheless, the emergence of faith in the Trinity at the dawn of the Christian era is a remarkable phenomenon, and it may be possible to come to terms with some of the religious experience of the early Christians which led them to their faith in the triune God.

In the context of ancient Israel, the early Christian faith in the Trinity is quite amazing. For thousands of years the Jewish people had struggled toward monotheism, toward the purging of all beliefs in false gods, and toward a commitment to the one God who is all holy. Surely this achievement of a radical monotheism is the great contribution of Judaism to the history of the world.[2] This makes it all the more surprising that the infant Christian church began to speak of the one God as a triune God. Just what was it in the early experience of the church which elicited the faith response to the Trinity? While we will never know completely, it seems at least reasonable to argue that the first Christians were so moved by Jesus' love for them that they simply could not conceive of God unless God were persons loving one another, unless God were somehow a community of persons in love. This ultimately is what our faith in the Trinity says: God, while utterly one, is persons in love and forming community with one another. Various theologians across the centuries have articulated this theme of the trinitarian God being utterly one, except for the community of relationships which exist in God. In our own century, this understanding of the Trinity has been expressed with particular eloquence by Karl Rahner.[3]

From this perspective, our trinitarian theology becomes a radical challenge to community. How can Christians say they believe in God if they are unwilling to put together structures that build human community and meet fundamental human needs? How can someone really claim to believe in the triune God and not feel a sense of outrage about the quarter of the U.S. population which lacks or is inadequately supplied with such a basic good as health care coverage? If we believe in the triune God as the very ground of community, the problem of our health care system is not just an ethical or economic or political problem. The problem is ultimately a religious or theological problem.

I have grounded the notion of God as radical community in the Christian mystery of God as Trinity. It seems, however, that other believers in God could come to an understanding of God as the source of community without a belief in the Trinity. Similarly, those who reject explicit faith in God but who have an open, meaning-centered view of life could come to a philosophy which argues that life itself calls us to form bonds with one another and build community.[4] The point is that the call to communal responsibility comes from the very core of life, rather than being a more peripheral aspect of human existence. Christians express this community-centered core through their faith in the Trinity, but this notion is accessible in various ways.

The other important thing about our faith in the Trinity is that, beyond the Trinity's communitarian implications, the Trinity must be understood as radical and holy mystery, as beyond our power to ever fully understand even in heaven. This theme of God as the inexpressible mystery has an important driving power to influence us as we look at issues like health care justice.[5] If God is radical mystery, then we never fully understand life and its future, we are not really sure just where we are going, we do not know what wonderful things God might have in store for us, not only in heaven but even here on earth.

To say this in another way, God's mysteriousness makes us a restless people, a people not quite satisfied with things the way they are, a people always looking for new options, a people hoping new hopes and dreaming new dreams. Some theologies of the past have tended to construe God as the one who keeps everything the way it is, the one who holds us together in being. There is no reason to deny the notion of God as the support and conservator of our existence, but the idea of God as the mover and shaker and the one who energizes us and pulls us into a new and uncharted future seems even more central to our faith in the triune God. Some would even argue that the best and truest way in which to speak of God is as our absolute future to which we surrender in faith and love.[6]

In the world of health care reform, this basic restlessness which comes from faith in the God who calls us to community can have a significant impact. When we look at the problems of health care today, how could we be anything other than restless? When we look at the problems, we also need to be willing to dream new dreams, and to let go of old idols such as "Massive government programs are the only answer" or "Government will automatically mess things up if it tries to do this or that." Only a radical theological hope and a radical theological care for one another can give us the core freedom we will need to move toward health care reform. In ways we do not usually think about, and in ways we will never completely understand, the hope, care, and freedom we need are grounded in our faith in God.

CHRIST AND THE CHURCH

While it has a crucial importance, the "God talk" of the last few paragraphs also has a certain abstractness. For Christians, the abstractness of God comes to an end with the incarnation, with the definitive entry of God into human history through the person of Jesus Christ. As the divine and the human intersect in Jesus, the questions of community and of care for one another become even more clearly focused. If there is any one feature which marks the life and ministry of Jesus, it is his love for people, his calling us together to be his beloved community. We see this in Jesus' care for his friends, people like Martha, Mary, Lazarus, Peter, John, Mary Magdalene, and so on. We see it in his words: "Love one another as I have loved you." "By this will all know that you are my disciples, that you love one another." "I no longer call you servants, but I call you friends." This last notion, that we are all friends in Christ, is the beginning of a theology of the church. In so many ways, this is what our faith is all about: being friends to one another as Jesus was friend to us. The human bonding which this friendship involves is the source of the claim mentioned earlier in the book, the claim that calls us to watch and keep company with one another as we face our own sickness and dying. Being sick and dying are things we cannot do very well alone. To be sick and die well we need to be a community of friends sharing a covenant of love with one another.

If Jesus' life and ministry are in a special way a statement about love and friendship, I think it is particularly fascinating that many of Jesus' friendships were with sick people, and that so much of his ministry was to people who needed healing. We can think about Peter's mother-in-law, about the paralytic who was lowered through the roof, about the man born blind, about the royal official's son, about Lazarus, and many others. This is not the place to review the scriptural problems which surround some of the miracle stories in the gospels. Regardless of those problems, the point is that Jesus' ministry was very specially a ministry of friendship and healing. I think the call to a deep community bonding around health care issues should be clear to all who would call themselves followers of Jesus.

Out of Jesus' life of love and community, there sprung his community of love, the church. Here we will not discuss all the questions about the exact character of the founding of the church by Jesus. Instead, we will review four themes which help to focus the nature of the church as a community of love, a community which calls us to establish meaningful social structures. The four themes will be the church as the people of God, as a covenantal love community, as the source of sacramental life, and as an organized institution.

When I first applied to the seminary in the late 1950s, I was interviewed by a wonderful older priest who helped the bishop decide which candidates to accept. Most potential candidates, myself included, received a little advance priming for the interview from the priests in their own parishes. One crucially important point was this: when you were asked why you wanted to be a priest, the first answer should be that you wanted to be a priest in order to save your own soul. After having said that, you could go on to say that you also hoped you might be able to help other individuals save their own souls. Needless to say, I answered the questions in the accepted manner. I had little doubt about the validity of the answers because in those days "saving your own soul" was to a large extent what the church seemed to be all about, not only for prospective seminarians, but for many others.

This earlier theology of saving your individual soul has relatively little communitarian emphasis. But beginning in the 1940s, Pope Pius XII began to stress the idea that the church is the body of Christ.[7] Even more importantly, Vatican II, in its great document *Lumen Gentium,* taught that perhaps the best way to understand the church is to see the church as the people of God,[8] as the assembly of believers gathered together with the common mission of supporting and sharing with all people. In the years since Vatican II, the people of God theme has had a great impact on Catholic life so that many parishes and other Catholic institutions are much more truly communities of faith than they were at one time.

In our present context the point of this community-based ecclesiology is that we must move from a "get your own health needs taken care of" mentality to a sense of communal responsibility for the health of all people. While not as many Catholics today would make "saving my soul" their primary language, it is not clear how much the more communitarian theology of church has worked its way into the thinking of Catholics and other U.S. citizens about health care.

Another rich biblical theme which helps shape our understanding of the church as community is the theme of covenant, the theme that God calls us together as a community of love rooted in God. Over and over again, the scriptures remind us of God's love covenant with us: "I will be your God and you will be my people." Covenant language reminds us of the radical seriousness with which we must take other people; it reminds us of that deeper love and loyalty which we owe to one another because of our shared faith and because of our common humanity. In many areas of life today there is a tendency to say that relationships between human beings are strictly business, that bonded covenant love need not enter in. Even in health care, the business aspect of relationships can sometimes predominate so that the idea of covenant love becomes diminished. Hence the church's call to base relationships with one another on the theme of covenant is especially pertinent to the area of health care. Because health is so central to what human life is all about, how could a people of faith not see the health care needs of one another in terms of communal covenantal responsibilities?

Across the centuries, one of the most interesting aspects of the covenant love theme has been the issue of strangers, travelers, guests, or foreigners, and how we are especially called to reach out to such persons to give them our welcome, our hospitality. The famous Old Testament story of Sodom and Gomorrah has important connections with these hospitality traditions. The rule of St. Benedict (which saved for us so many values from the ancient world) has a wonderful section on the need to welcome pilgrim monks, coupled with a realism that over time the welcome can have some limitations.[9] It is fascinating to consider that the very word "hospital" springs from this venerable tradition of welcoming strangers in covenantal love.[10] While there are good reasons (because of the presence of so many out-patient services and doctor's offices), it is ironic that some hospitals today are dropping the word "hospital" from their official names. It is to be hoped that such name changes do not belie an understanding which focuses on the hospital more as a business entity than as a community where we are drawn together through the experience of God's faithful covenant love for us.

These reflections on the mission and ministry of the church very quickly bring to mind the sacramental life of the church. From the beginning the church has known that it cannot execute its mission of love in purely private or interior terms. Instead, the Catholic tradition has insisted on visible sacramental rites as an essential part of its mission and ministry. The church's insistence on the sacraments can be said to stem from the incarnational principle, i.e. from the awareness that we as humans live in time, space, and history. Because of our historical nature, religious experience can never be simply a "me and God" sort of affair. Religious experience is a public reality, it belongs to the community as a whole, it is to be celebrated by the community. The sacraments say that community really matters, that as believers we must care for one another in a visible and structured fashion.

In this context it should come as no surprise that many Catholic religious communities have had a notable historic involvement in the delivery of health care. Indeed it seems almost inevitable that a religion which has a high commitment to the sacramental principle would seek after organized involvement in health care. Our faith is a public or communal reality, and health care is one of the most central of all the areas of human need. Incarnationalism, which drives us to take our faith into the public area, is, after all, about embodiment. It is our bodies which make our spirituality public and sacramental. No wonder then that human needs which relate to embodiment and to the public character of life stand out as such a moral challenge to a sacramental faith community. Caring about the state of health care—for everyone, not just for oneself—is an expression of a sacramental life of faith.

Traditionally, the Catholic emphasis on sacrament has led to the establishment and maintenance of health care facilities. Today it can be argued that establishment and maintenance alone are not enough. In addition, the Catholic communal commitment to health care calls for advocacy, for public witness to the kind of reforms which are necessary to bring about just health care delivery. Such advocacy and calls for reform are a natural expression of the church's sacramental mission.[11]

One more point: While the sacraments make us think about public community witness, they also make us think about beauty. The sacraments say that the public character of our faith in God is to be celebrated in a manner which reflects the beauty and wonder of life. From this perspective, it seems that the Catholic community's efforts for health care reform ought to be committed to beauty and all that it entails.[12] For the Catholic, it is not enough simply to work for access to health care. Catholicism is also by its nature concerned that health care be delivered in a setting which is as humanly serene and respectful as possible. The pace of life for health care deliverers can be extraordinarily frenetic at times. But practices which shout out against our human sensibilities—like leaving patients naked for everyone who walks by to see—are to be avoided if at all possible. This may not be the most pivotal issue in health care reform, but reform will be all the more whole if a more just system of health care can be moved by a sense of beauty and avoid such aesthetic insensibilities.[13]

In the last few paragraphs, I have tried to show that, even though the church cares deeply for the dignity and worth of each individual person, it is the very nature of the church to be a community. Someone who comes from a church perspective cannot adopt the individualism which marks much of today's health care system. But just what kind of community is the church? How does it feel about matters such as organization, structure, law, etc.? How does it relate its views on organization and structure to the freedom of the individual? The answers to these questions can have an important impact on the specific type of health care reform which the church would be most likely to support.

To speak about the kind of organized community life which marks Roman Catholicism, we need to consider the sociology of religion. While there are many important works in this field, the pioneering work in religious sociology was done by the great German scholar Ernst Troeltsch at the beginning of the twentieth century. As Troeltsch saw it, the various Christian denominations can be divided into two main types: churches and sects.[14] Churches, according to Troeltsch, believe in visibly structured organizational patterns with clear rules and organized leadership. Churches typically relate closely to the world around them. Churches are interested in having large numbers of members and they are very likely to have infant baptism as a means of developing a large membership which can have an impact on the life of the world as a whole.

Sectarian Christian groups on the other hand tend to base themselves much more on the charismatic inspirations of individual members. They are less interested in organized structures and policies and they may very well not have authoritative patterns of leadership. Voluntary commitment is much more the basis for the existence of the sects. In their concern for the individual holiness of their members, sects are much more likely to have adult baptism. Their membership will be stronger because they only want truly committed members. Sects often see themselves as very distant from the world and its problems. Some sects even drop out of the organized political world as we know it.[15]

While there may be no Christian denomination which is an exactly perfect fit in Troeltsch's church/sect paradigm, Troeltsch certainly seems to be on the mark in his depiction of the two major patterns of church organization. It is important to remember also that there are valuable aspects to both church-type bodies and sectarian-type bodies. Church types have the advantage of being interested in the world around them which creates the potential for bringing about meaningful reforms. But church types can be so close to the world and its "conventional wisdom" that they can fail to see serious social problems or fail to imagine any truly creative solutions to these problems. Sectarians on the other hand are often much freer from the pressures of conventional society. Historically they have been among the first to see the social problems involved in slavery, prison management, modern warfare systems, etc. But sectarians can get so distant from the world that they are ineffectual as agents for social change.

It should be obvious that, in Troeltsch's terms, Roman Catholicism understands itself much more as a church than as a sect. With some differences, groups such as Anglicans, Presbyterians, and Lutherans also belong to the church category. In such groups, structure, organization, and law are part of the commitment to community and community building. This is important in the context of health care reform because groups with a church orientation are much less likely to think that health care reform can be accomplished through efforts which are largely or completely voluntary. Instead, the church approach to community would more naturally think of law and authoritative government activity as an essential part of the health care reform. Ever since 1919 the Roman Catholic Church in the United States has been actively involved in efforts for social reform through meaningful legislation.[16] Such efforts began with the work of Msgr. John A. Ryan and have continued all the way to the bishops' recent pastorals on nuclear arms and economic justice. The Catholic approach to community entails a commitment to public social reform.

There is an interesting and ironic side note here, namely that while Roman Catholicism is clearly a church in the Troeltschian sense, Roman Catholicism contains within it many religious orders or communities whose histories are often rather like the histories of the various Christian sects. Nor is it surprising that the church's strong historic commitment to health care has been largely under the sponsorship of these religious communities with their greater freedom to be aware of changing social needs. It may be that in the approach to health care reform, Catholicism will be able to bring both something of the church order outlook with its commitment to effective social structures and something of the sectarian critical outlook with its passion for meaningful change. If so, the Catholic communal approach to health care reform can be all the stronger.

Another point to be noted in this context is that Christian groups with sectarian origins are growing more and more prominent in U.S. society today. This is especially the case with biblical fundamentalist groups. I have no doubt at all about the genuine Christian convictions of such groups. But it may be that their views on the nature of community will be less apt to serve as a basis for the structured social change which may be necessary for health care reform. This could be all the more reason for the Catholic Church and other "churches" to bring their resources to bear in the debate about health care reform.

In Chapter 7 we will focus on the question of what the church and the theologians have to say on health care reform in comparison to the views of economists, politicians, health care professionals, etc. Here our focus was on the nature of church community and on how different approaches to church community would have different impacts on the approach to health care reform.

THE INDIVIDUAL BELIEVER AND COMMUNITY BUILDING

If God, Christ, and the church have about them an essential community building orientation and an awareness of the need for organized social structures, what about the individual believer? Can the believer see his or her faith in purely private terms, in terms which focus exclusively on a "save my own soul" approach to faith? These questions might be approached in various ways, but if we accept the idea that the love of God is the crowning point of the Christian life, it might help to look at the whole meaning of love from a faith perspective.

It is of course commonplace to assert that love of neighbor and love of God go together. As scripture puts it, "How can we love the God whom we cannot see, unless we love our neighbor whom we can see?" (1 Jn 4:20). But why is this so? Why can't we have a purely private love of God? What sort of religious anthropology serves as the foundation for the idea that the love of God and the love of neighbor are inextricably intertwined?

As soon as we acknowledge that God is totally spiritual and that we humans are embodied or incarnate spirits, we must face the fact that as humans we can never know and love God except in and through knowing and loving one another. Our spirituality is frozen in our materiality.[17] Only concrete tangible experiences can open our spirituality, can make us aware of God. Thomas Aquinas asserted this clearly in the middle ages when he said that all knowledge begins with sense knowledge.[18] It is true of course that many kinds of concrete experience are possible for the human person. But the high point of concrete human experience is the experience of other persons. It is for this reason that the act of love of neighbor is the supreme tangible expression of human love for God. In the final analysis it can be said that every act of loving God is at the same time an act of loving other human persons and vice versa.[19] For humans it is a contradiction in terms to say that we can love God without loving other human persons. This is not to claim that there is only one way to love other people. Our love for God can be expressed through various kinds of human love.

When we speak about this theological aspect of human love, we are speaking about the concrete historical nature of human persons. Hence we should reject the idea that our love for other people can be limited to romance and personal friendships, as important as these can be. Rather we are talking about love for people in the world as it actually exists, love in a world which has an organized history in which politics and economics are very real. From a theological viewpoint, the love of neighbor must involve a care for the world, a care for its structures, a care for justice. Otherwise our love would be empty and vacuous. It would not really be love for God.

It is fascinating to note that from the viewpoint of theology, the concrete historical character of human love is rooted in the reality of human embodiment. This suggests that genuine human love ought to care about our embodiment and about everything related to it. Sometimes people wonder why the church is concerned about issues like housing, hunger, the rights of prisoners and immigrants, etc. All these issues relate to our embodied human needs and thus are very appropriate focus points for Christian love and care. Health care needs relate with unique closeness to our embodiment. This makes health care and the reform of health care delivery a very natural object for Christian love of neighbor. If the love of God by definition calls us to love and care for one another, there are few more loving things we can do than to provide for people's reasonable health care needs. All this will be considered further in the next chapter which will reflect on health care as a human right.

Another point of significance is that, while Christian love can take many worthwhile forms, our tradition is that the highest form of Christian love is the love known as agape, the love of other people for their own sake, love which expects no return. The earmark of agape love is that it is a love which sets other people free, free to grow and develop independently of the persons who are giving the love. If it is true that health problems can entrap human persons and limit their freedom, then it is also true that providing for people's genuine health care needs can be a very freeing expression of love. Martin Luther King was fond of saying that as the people of God we are called to build a "beloved community" here on earth.[20] There seems little doubt that health care reform can be a major part of that Christian love which builds community.

The case for the individual person as community builder can also be argued by pointing to the Christian concept of grace which holds that if we are in true union with God, the very life of God flows within us. Some authors speak about God's grace as divinizing us, as making the communal love of the Trinity the core of our existence.[21] Here I chose to emphasize the theme of love because of its action-oriented links to our neighbors. But the theology of grace also connects to the same basic concerns.

NATURAL LAW: BUILDING JUST COMMUNITY HERE ON EARTH

In the past few sections we have asserted that our faith in God, Christ, and the church calls us to be loving community builders who act for meaningful social change. But the Christian tradition is more than theology alone. Especially in Roman Catholicism, there has been much disciplined philosophical thinking on the natural character of human community and government. We now turn our attention to some key points from Catholic philosophy, beginning with the natural law tradition.

The notion of natural law originated with ancient Greek thinkers such as Aristotle and with ancient Roman stoicism. After centuries of absence from scholarly awareness, the theme of natural law was recovered in the middle ages shortly before the time of Thomas Aquinas who had so much to do with revitalizing the natural law tradition.[22] Unfortunately, many people associate the term "natural law" with a set of specific regulations about personal moral issues, especially issues related to sexuality. Actually, natural law has a much deeper meaning. It refers to the fact that God created the world as a moral world in which there is an inherent difference between right and wrong. Natural law also refers to the shared capacity of human persons to know the difference between right and wrong, at least for the most part. This capacity to know right from wrong exists on the basis of our very humanity, not because of God's revelation in the scriptures, so that all people in all eras and cultures share in the gift of natural law even when they have to struggle to work out its specific implications (as we obviously do in the area of health care justice). Finally, natural law refers to the fact that our knowledge of right and wrong is not merely theoretical. We experience ourselves as obligated to do what is good and to avoid evil.

This notion of natural law as a basic capacity of human persons for moral living is suggested more clearly in some other languages than it is in English. The French speak about *le droit natural* and the Germans speak of *naturecht*, with both of these terms suggesting something along the line of natural moral rights or claims which we have upon one another. The Latin often speaks about *ius naturale* which we might translate as a natural capacity for justice.

As these terms suggest, natural law, whatever limitations some of its historical expressions might have had, is a philosophy with a high faith in the human person's potential for goodness. Because of this potential, the natural law tradition is convinced that human community is possible, that it is possible for us to live together here on this planet, that it is possible for us to understand and act on the basis of meaningful shared standards of human behavior. In the natural law context, the possibility of communal moral standards means that government can be an enabler of the good for all people.[23] Government does not exist simply because we are evil and need protection from one another's wickedness. Nor does government exist so that those who have faith can impose their religious beliefs on others. Rather government exists because strong and deeply bonded human community is possible here on earth and government can serve as a creative agency to enhance such community. Earlier I spoke about the U.S. Catholic bishops' articulate support for government policies of social reform throughout the twentieth century. Once we take note of Catholic thought's powerful roots in the natural law tradition, and of natural law's belief in structured human community, the historic role of the bishops comes as no surprise.

Due to the power and importance of the natural law tradition, I was somewhat troubled by the questions about natural law which came up during the first Clarence Thomas hearings. Whatever one thinks about Thomas himself, the questions about natural law seemed to imply that our public policies are purely arbitrary government creations. The idea that there are higher moral standards to which any government is bound seemed absent in the questions about natural law. The U.S. Constitution is after all a human instrument. There have been and will be times when it is legitimately changed and challenged on the basis of a growing understanding of fundamental human rights issues.

I have often thought that if the natural law tradition did not exist we would have to invent it in order to make human living practical. For example, how could any human community be possible if we thought that human persons did not share an understanding of the importance of telling the truth? If we thought that people were just as likely to lie to us as to tell us the truth, how could we ever believe or trust anybody? If the food or drugs we buy are as likely to be tainted as to be pure, wouldn't we all need to go back to working our own little farms, and wouldn't this mean that many of the wonderful accomplishments of civilization would have to be abandoned?

Sadly, we do know that sometimes people will lie, steal, cheat, and commit murder. We know that government needs to enact sanctions against such misbehaviors and at least in part serves to protect us from one another's sins. But if it is true that most people most of the time try to do what is right, then human community truly becomes possible. Even in those areas where we are not sure what the answers are, the positive community spirit at the heart of the natural law tradition says we can keep on talking with one another, working with one another, and experimenting with different approaches to justice until we find the most reasonable answer to a problem. As Reinhold Niebuhr was fond of saying, our pilgrim status here on earth will mean that sometimes our answer will be a second-best answer or a proximate solution.[24] But a second-best solution is often a good solution, surely better than no solution at all.

It is important to remember that natural law is not a perfect system. Many critics feel that it is too focused on personal moral issues such as sexual conduct standards to be an effective enabler of meaningful social policies. This criticism rings true for some particular interpretations of natural law, but I do not think it is fair to the heart of the natural law tradition. More significantly, natural law is limited when it comes to working out all the details of difficult moral problems. We cannot claim that it will give us easy answers to issues such as health care justice. The Catholic bishops of the U.S. showed an excellent awareness of the limits of particular applications of natural law in their pastoral letter on nuclear arms.[25] Such an awareness ought to mark all of our thinking about natural law.

A perspective on these criticisms can be gained by noting that over the past few decades many Protestant scholars have begun to assert the importance of natural law as a foundation for shared dialogue about difficult human problems. Because of Protestant theology's historic opposition to natural law, some of these more recent Protestant scholars have proposed alternative terms to describe natural law, with John Coleman Bennett's "common ground morality" being a well-known example of an alternative term.[26] Whatever terms are used, natural law has a broader base of ecumenical support than in the past.

In the specific context of health care reform, it would surely be wrong to claim that natural law can give us an easy set of solutions to the crisis we face. The multiplicity of proposals we looked at in Chapter 2 make it obvious that the specifics of health care reform will not come about easily. But natural law's basic assumption—that we live in a shared moral universe where there are values to be held in common—makes it seem possible to keep working toward a truly communal approach to health care justice. With natural law, there is a ground for hope, a ground for continued dialogue about health care justice, a basis for trusting that with our common humanity we can move together to a health care system which is at least reasonable if not perfect. Because of our limited and fallible human learning processes, many of the moral goods we seek are unknowns yet to be known or discovered. In natural law philosophy, there is the hope that the unknown yet to be known can be discovered, even in a difficult area like health care justice. Our moral capacities are not isolated from one another. The search for social justice remains a genuine possibility.

A CATHOLIC PHILOSOPHY OF CIVIL LAW

These comments about natural law have underlined the human capacity to keep struggling with difficult moral issues such as health care justice. But what about the role of specific civil legislation as an enabler of a more just health care system? Would the Catholic natural law outlook suggest that dialogue and community-building should take place only on a private sector basis? Or would legislative action be an appropriate way to build moral community in the health care sector? It should come as no surprise that Catholicism, with its belief in sacraments, institutions, and natural law, would have a favorable view on the role of legislation in promoting social change.

To explain this more specifically, it is interesting to note the legal philosophy of Martin Luther. He held that laws existed for two purposes: to remind us of our sinfulness and to maintain civil order. In the Latin, Luther's first use of law is called the *usus condemnatus,* and his second use is called the *usus civilis.* From this Lutheran perspective, civil government stands as a "dike against sin," or as the "left hand of God." All this is part of Luther's famous two-realm theory in which the church is a law-free realm based on goodness while the state exists in a law-based realm to deal with the problem of sin.[27]

In the classic understanding of Luther's approach, civil government protects us from those who would do us harm. But civil government has no role in enacting legislation to try to enhance the human condition. Civil government is so marked by sin that any laws it enacts to improve our lot will be sin-tainted and ultimately useless.[28] This view would hold that defense, with its protective character, is an appropriate government task. But legislation to promote social reform is not a suitable government task. It seems fair to say that several of the recent U.S. administrations have had a rather Lutheran outlook on their role, an outlook without strong interest in health care reform. It should also be said that many Lutheran theologians have developed carefully nuanced versions of this famous Lutheran approach. Not all Lutheran theology is totally one-sided in its views of law and social reform.

John Calvin accepted Luther's two uses of law, but in his writings he also added a third and even more central use for law. Calvin felt that first and foremost law can serve to teach us how to live as a better community of persons here on earth. This is the use of law as a pedagogue (*usus pedagogicus*).[29] In asserting the role of law as a teacher, Calvin, while not forgetting the problem of human sinfulness, took a position similar to that of Thomas Aquinas, meaning that both the Roman Catholic tradition and the Presbyterian tradition have had a much more positive understanding of the role of government as an enactor of legislation aimed at bringing about the human good. In these religious traditions, legislation to deal with the health care crisis would be seen as a perfectly normal and coherent task for government.

There is an interesting scholarly debate on the relative merits of Catholicism and Calvinism as philosophies of social change. Some scholars hold that, because of Thomas' strong belief in the goodness of the social order, Catholicism is more cautious about social change out of concern not to upset the good which already exists. The same scholars would argue that Calvinism is somewhat more ready to opt for radical social change, both out of a strong sense that sin needs to be challenged and out of a sense of God's dynamism breaking into human history. The work of H. Richard Niebuhr was especially helpful in trying to articulate these slight differences between the two traditions.[30] In our next chapter when we consider the notion of the common good, we will need to look at all this in more detail. Here we need not resolve all areas of difference between those churches who believe that public legislation can be used to better the human condition. Our point is that Catholicism and other important segments of the Christian tradition are convinced of the place of law as an enabler of social change and social justice. Some in the U.S. seem to have rejected this positive sense of law as the builder of community. Recovery of this traditional Catholic/Calvinist sense of law seems essential for true health care reform.

In these comments about law we have not dealt with two issues. First, even though the Roman Catholic tradition clearly supports civil law as a means of bringing about social reform, Catholicism by no means rules out voluntary initiative as a means to social change. So just what sort of blending of civil law and voluntary effort is the best way to build a moral community? Second, while it is clear that Catholicism believes that institutions, governments, and laws can build the human community, how exactly does Catholicism understand the common good which governments, laws, and institutions should seek to build? In both of these questions we begin to move from the fundamental theological/philosophical vision of community toward the matter of the more explicitly ethical character of our communal life. These and other questions will form the main focus of our next chapter.

VIRTUE AND THE BUILDING OF COMMUNITY

Very often when we think about an issue such as health care reform, we think about particular decisions which will need to be made to put health care reform in place. While such particular decisions are both important and necessary in all areas of moral concern, including health care, such decisions do not capture the whole of what we are called to be about as a religious/moral community. In addition to individual decisions, the call to community involves the practice of moral living, involves ongoing day-to-day habits with which we reach out to one another with love and care. Almost inevitably, our efforts at health care reform will not be fully successful at first, meaning that people will need to persevere in an ongoing struggle for a more just system.

This notion that our communal life comes out of the practice of community, out of habits of community, is usually described by saying that community life depends on virtuous people, i.e. people committed to living out true community life day after day and year after year. In traditional Roman Catholic thought, the theology of the virtuous life occupied a major place. In earlier times, no student of Catholic moral theology would have made it through the curriculum without taking at least one extended course on the virtues. It is regrettable that the virtues are not more emphasized in Roman Catholic theological education in our own times.

The importance of virtue and character as sources of community has been emphasized in more recent years by philosophers such as Alasdair McIntyre in his *After Virtue*,[31] by Protestant theologians such as Stanley Hauerwas in books such as *A Community of Character*,[32] and by sociologists such as Robert Bellah and his co-authors in the highly significant work *Habits of the Heart*.[33] McIntyre and Hauerwas retrieve some of the best of Aristotle and Aquinas while Bellah and his co-authors proceed from an analysis of U.S. life today. In all these authors, the challenge is clear that we can only build community on the basis of the kind of people we are, not on legal policies or individual decisions taken out of context.

These thoughts suggest that we all have to work or practice at building community. Young people are not born fully prepared to be community builders. They need to learn the skills, the virtues, the habits. The role of parents, educators, clergy, public officials, and other similar models is crucially important, especially in an era when the hero worship of sports and entertainment figures is so predominant, even though very few young people will ever succeed in playing these roles.

In the health care world, all this means that in the quest for justice there will be an ever growing need for great doctors, great nurses, great administrators, great social workers and pastoral caregivers, and so on. These people will need to be great not simply in terms of their professional skills but in terms of their steady virtuous human caring. If they are great in this way, they can draw other gifted people into the world of health care. This can make the health care world into a true community where genuine reform may at last be possible.

The communal virtue of which I speak depends significantly on good stories, stories about true heroism in the delivery of health care. In Baltimore, the Sisters at Mercy Medical Center still remember how their predecessors helped and cared for the firefighters in the great Baltimore fire of 1904. Today's firefighters and police also remember, so that almost a century later there still exists a special spirit of co-operation which is so helpful for the workings of an inner city hospital which often has to deal with difficult situations involving groups like firefighters and police personnel. No doubt there are similar stories elsewhere, stories which serve as a school for virtue and for the building of true community.

These comments about virtue and community bring us to the end of this exploration of some of the religious and philosophical roots of community. Surely other community generating factors could also be cited. But hopefully it is clear that we cannot think about the ethics of health care delivery only in terms of individual patients and their individual care needs. Unless we see ourselves, both religiously and humanly, as called to true community, adequate health care reform will be a dream. True community may call for some sacrifices, some giving up of individual hopes in the area of health care. But how can tomorrow's health care be just, other than as community health care?

Chapter 6

THE ETHICS OF THE
JUST COMMUNITY AND
THE REFORM OF HEALTH CARE

We turn now to the most substantive questions in this book, the questions about the moral obligation of the just community to bring about health care reform. For me it was very important not to treat these questions without first setting up the context of the theology of the person and the community. But the justice questions are crucially significant, and it is time to try to address them directly. Many sources will be called upon as we look at the justice questions, but there will be a special emphasis on the social teaching of the Catholic Church since 1891.

This chapter will consider five main issues about the just community and health care: first, human rights and health care; second, the common good as the basis for health care delivery; third, distributive justice and the delivery of health care; fourth, the ethics of health care rationing; fifth, the relationship between government action and private action in the delivery of health care, with particular emphasis on the question of how the principles of subsidiarity and socialization interact in the field of health care.

In terms of the logic of Roman Catholic theology, it might have been more coherent to place the treatment of human rights after the sections on the common good and the meaning of distributive justice. However, since so much of the twentieth century debate about just health care has focused on the notion of a human right to health care, it seemed most useful to treat this issue first and then to critically develop our understanding of health care rights as we consider the subsequent and even more foundational material on the common good and on justice.

HUMAN RIGHTS AND HEALTH CARE

To address the issue of human rights and health care, we will look at three themes: the historical development of the human rights tradition, some of the current critiques of human rights thinking, and the specific question of whether persons have a right to a basic level of health care.

THE MODERN HISTORY OF HUMAN RIGHTS

Secular Political Developments

Historically, human rights thinking has developed on both a secular political track and a religious or theological track. In the secular or political arena, we usually think of the major emphasis on human rights as having begun with the French Declaration of the Rights of Man (1789) and the U.S. Bill of Rights (1790). These two documents espouse what is often called the liberal theory of human rights, i.e. the right of persons not to be interfered with as they pursue their goals in life. This level of human rights thinking fits in well with the individualistic thinking of the philosopher John Locke, and with the laissez faire economics of Adam Smith. Sometimes we call the rights in our Bill of Rights civil rights or political rights. Whatever the exact language, the thinking behind the liberal theory of human rights has a certain negative quality about it. These rights are rights to be left on one's own, rights to immunity from harm. Government's tasks are to pass laws guaranteeing these rights and to be sure that no one acts against us to take these rights away. But beyond these tasks, government does not have to organize any programs to provide these rights to people.

Hidden within the liberal theory of human rights is a fairly high awareness of the problem of human sin.[1] No one ought to be allowed to interfere with our liberty, because with our common sinfulness, none of us is wise enough to place limits on the liberty of others. If government tries to do more than protect us from one another and from outsiders, government will inevitably mess things up. It is ironic that this viewpoint historically has been called "the liberal view." Today we tend to call persons with this right outlook "conservative," and we use the word "liberal" in very different contexts.

Surely we can make some criticisms of the classic liberal view of human rights. We might argue, for example, that the classic liberal view offers little basis for any assertion of a right to health care. However, when we stop to consider that, before the time of the French and American revolutions, many persons' lives were rigidly controlled by repressive political regimes, it is clear that the emphasis on personal freedom did much to advance our awareness of the dignity and worth of each human person. This emphasis on dignity and freedom is an important part of the overall human rights tradition, with significant links to the issue of why all people should have access to basic health care.

In the mid-nineteenth century, another level of human rights thinking began to emerge in the secular political sphere. This level was not so much concerned with protecting our freedom from outside interference. Instead this level was concerned with what steps government and society might be able to take to positively enhance our condition as human persons. Unlike the earlier liberal tradition with its concern for civil rights, this later political tradition began to speak about social and economic rights. Today we sometimes use the terms "entitlements" and "welfare rights" to describe the social and economic rights which are at issue. Marxist and socialist thinkers were prominent in the early thinking about economic and social rights, but the concern for socio-economic rights is by no means limited to Marxists and socialists. Anyone who advocates some kind of "mixed economy" (in which capitalism operates under certain social controls) is concerned about social rights.[2]

When we stop to think about it we can easily see that there is a tension between the liberal theory of civil rights and the emphasis on socio-economic rights. Those who would emphasize socio-economic rights sometimes argue in favor of limiting certain civil rights (e.g. the right to free enterprise) in order to provide basic economic rights to all people. Public life in the United States is currently based on a compromise between the two theories of human rights, with one side stressing liberty and the other equality. The differing proposals for health care reform which we reviewed in Chapter 2 have different slants on human rights. Some of them are more interested in keeping free enterprise and the liberal view of rights in the primary position, while other proposals are more convinced of the need to limit individual rights so as to advance social rights in the area of health care.

Roman Catholic Thinking on Rights

Earlier we saw that, in following Aristotle, Thomas Aquinas had a fairly positive notion of the responsibility of government to enhance human dignity. In addition, during the nineteenth century Catholic leaders were becoming very much aware of the growing social problems caused by the industrial revolution. For these reasons, it is not surprising that when modern Catholic social teaching began with Pope Leo XIII's *Rerum Novarum* (1891), there was a significant emphasis on the social side of human rights. Probably the most famous section of *Rerum Novarum* is Pope Leo's call for all working persons to be paid a living wage.[3] While Pope Leo did speak very briefly about human rights, he placed greater stress on the duties and responsibilities which are correlative to human rights. None of this, however, means that Pope Leo endorsed socialism or Marxism. His arguments in *Rerum Novarum* in favor of private property are very conservative from an economic point of view.[4] He managed to combine a concern for socio-economic rights with a rather traditional view of economics.

Pope Leo XIII's conservative outlook gave him a mistrust of nineteenth century liberalism, especially in France. He believed in the importance of stable governments, and he worried that too much stress on individual civil liberties might serve to undermine governments. Thus it seems fair to say that, unlike modern secular political thought, which began with liberal rights and then moved to social rights, modern Catholic social thought began with a greater emphasis on social rights and only later moved to a stronger emphasis on civil rights.

With Pope Leo's encyclical as a benchmark, I think it can be said that twentieth century Roman Catholic thought on human rights has seen three important developments beyond Pope Leo's teaching. First, and most important, there has been a reassessment of the types of economic policies which might be used to assure human rights. Private ownership, which Pope Leo saw as critically necessary, is no longer the only acceptable means to bring about the delivery of human rights. In 1931 Pope Pius XI continued the church's clear rejection of the atheism and materialism which is often part of the socialist approach to life. But at the same time, Pius XI began to assert that, at some times in history, the economic power of some businesses and groups in society may need to be regulated by government in order to bring about human rights.[5] This sort of thinking became even more explicit in later popes such as Paul VI with his call for the break-up of the great landed estates in Latin America.[6] In his encyclical *Sollicitudo Rei Socialis* (1988), Pope John Paul II seems to be quite even-handed in his criticism of both capitalism and socialism as economic systems.[7] In view of this trend in Roman Catholic thought, it would seem that, whatever their pros and cons, none of the major proposals for health care reform can be stated to be in clear opposition to Catholic social teaching.

A second trend in twentieth century Roman Catholic rights think-ing has been the growing emphasis on the dignity of the human person, so that individual rights such as freedom, participation, and self-expression have become substantially more present in Catholic teaching. This concern, which was seen as early as Pope Pius XII, became especially prominent in Pope John XXIII's famous encyclical *Pacem in Terris*[8] and in Vatican II's *Declaration on Religious Liberty*.[9] Through the writing of these popes, Catholicism has become gradu-ally less hierarchical in its view of society, and more accepting of the ethos of many of the modern democratic states. The themes of per-sonal freedom and participation may have significant potential for helping us shape contemporary approaches to health care reform. These themes can help us be more aware of the dignity of the poor and the sick. In addition, the clearer Catholic emphasis on the civil and political side of human rights may help Catholic hospitals to main-tain their legitimate autonomy.

Finally and briefly, in the twentieth century, Roman Catholic rights thinking can be said to have become more theological in its focus and less based on philosophy and ethics alone. In this context it is hard not to think of the World Synod of Bishops' famous 1971 assertion that action in behalf of social justice is a constitutive dimen-sion of preaching the gospel.[10] There are important debates about how to interpret this statement,[11] but its focus clearly makes the hu-man rights debate more of a religious issue than it once was.

Current Critiques of Human Rights

On the whole, the human rights tradition has a very important history both politically and religiously. Recently, however, I have be-gun to notice in some of my students a level of dissatisfaction with human rights as an ethical issue. These students are saying that they think human rights has become too much of an individualistic, me-against-you, category of thought. Statements such as "I demand my rights" seem not to suggest a wholistic or communal approach to who we are for one another as a community of persons. In the context of health care delivery too much insistence on what someone thinks is his or hers by right may obscure efforts to establish a common framework about what we can and cannot do in the health care arena. We saw earlier that most of the accomplishments of the progressive and rather successful Canadian health care system have been due to the efficiency of the system's design. But so far Canada's use of global budgeting has meant that the harder questions about Canada's health priorities as a nation have not yet been asked in the deepest sense, i.e. the questions of which health care services Canada should and should not offer all its citizens based on a common set of moral principles. Such questions may not be able to be asked exclusively on the basis of the human rights tradition, especially when this tradition is construed in its more individualistic forms.

Some recent scholarship has helped point out the limitations of the human rights model of ethical thinking. In her book *Rights Talk: The Impoverishment of Political Discourse,* Harvard law professor Mary Anne Glendon argues that an over-concern for individual rights can serve to rob us of a strong sense of the common good.[12] Listening to her critique it is hard not to think back to Pope Leo XIII a century ago with his fears about human rights thinking. Of course no one today would want to endorse the very static and hierarchical view of society which marked Pope Leo's thought. But his concern for the excess of individualism which can mark human rights thinking has a clear relevance today.

I would not argue that these critiques should cause us to abandon the human rights tradition, particularly in the area of health care. There is a positive and necessary importance in our reflecting on the claims or expectations which each of us has from one another and from society. But it is increasingly clear that rights language needs to be balanced with the language of duties, responsibilities, and communal concerns. It is also clear that the idea of rights as immunities or protections from harm needs to be balanced with the idea of rights as welfare rights or entitlements.

A Right to Health Care

Based on the human rights tradition can we say that persons have a right to health care? To begin our answer, several clarifications must be made, both linguistic and historical. Linguistically, it is to be emphasized that we are not speaking about a right to health, because so much of our health is dependent on our genetic make-up and other similar factors over which society has no control. Some would say that we do have a right not to have our health interfered with by environmental pollution or other similar influences, but even this kind of protection will not assure that everyone will be in good health. No one can guarantee this, even though some in our society seem to expect it and even though some facets of today's medicine (such as the defensiveness in medicine due to fear of lawsuits) exist because of the false expectations of a right to health. Also, in speaking of a right to health care, it is not adequate to speak about a right to any sort of health care whatsoever. Rather we are speaking about a right to a basic standard of health care.[13] Thus the precise rights question is whether persons can claim from society a basic standard of health care.

From the point of view of history, some might ask why health care has not been an issue for as long as human rights have been discussed. We saw earlier that when rights thinking first became politically prominent at the end of the eighteenth century, the focus was largely on civil rights, rights not to be interfered with. It is no surprise that health care was not considered among these non-interference rights. When social rights began to come to the fore in the mid-nineteenth century, medicine was still in a rather primitive state with relatively little good to offer. So here too it is not surprising that the early thinking about social rights did not place a high focus on health care as a human right. It was only in the last quarter of the nineteenth century that medicine (with the development of effective antiseptics and anesthetics by doctors such as Joseph Lister and Crawford Long) began to be able to offer the great goods which are so much a part of our consciousness today.[14] For this reason, the question of a basic standard of health care as a human right is largely a twentieth century question. Some countries such as Great Britain began to focus on this question in the early twentieth century, and many other countries faced the question in the middle part of the twentieth century. For the United States, the question remains very pressing as the twentieth century ends.[15]

But do all people have a right to basic access to health care at this time in human history? Ethically, I would argue yes for two main reasons. First, unlike earlier historical times, in our era basic access to health care can be a very great human good. Thus, if we accept the idea of social rights, it seems unthinkable not to include health care within those rights. Second, crises in health can happen to persons of all ages, economic conditions, degrees of social usefulness, etc. In other words, crises in health are part of our common humanity. We cannot tie these crises to any particular facet of our humanity so as to find a reasonable basis for limiting health care access to persons with non-medical human qualities such as virtue, usefulness, and wealth. It seems most just to see the need for health care as part of our common humanity, and thus to state that all persons, as human, have a right to an adequate level of health care. Rights language does have its limitations, but it still seems morally and religiously proper to speak of a human right to health care. Later in this chapter, our reflections on the common good and distributive justice will help further establish the notion of a basic or adequate level of health care as a human right.

The case that all persons have a right to a basic standard of health care seems to be coherent with recent official Roman Catholic teaching. In his famous encyclical *Pacem in Terris,* Pope John XXIII lists both medical care and security during sickness as elements in his listing of human rights.[16] In *Laborem Exercens,* Pope John Paul II speaks about the right of working people to health care which is cheap or even free.[17] I think it would be reasonable to extend the holy father's notion of cheap or free health care from working people to all people. In 1981 the Catholic bishops of the United States spoke of health care as "a basic human right which flows from the sanctity of human life."[18] In the Protestant world, the earlier General Assemblies of the World Council of Churches worked out of the notion of the "responsible society," a term with some Lockean roots, which may not have been as strongly open to a social right such as health care.[19] However, the more recent General Assemblies, beginning with Nairobi's emphasis on a "just, participatory, and sustainable society," have moved toward a more social focus on rights, a focus which appears open to the idea of a right to health care.[20] We should also note that Article 25 of the famous United Nations' Universal Declaration of Human Rights (1948) explicitly speaks both about a right to medical care and about a right to a standard of living adequate for the health and well-being of self and family.

In asserting the claim that all people have a right to an adequate level of health care, I have not addressed the issue of exactly what specific services should be included in this basic right. In Chapter 2 our review of current health care reform proposals showed a fair diversity on the specifics of what should be included. Certainly history will have its impact on the matter of the specifics because different services will be possible in different eras. Economics and medicine also have a lot to say about the specifics in terms of what it is feasible and beneficial to provide. In Chapter 8 I will present my own general outline of which types of services ought to be included in a just system of health care delivery. Here the point is more fundamental: to make the case that a basic standard of health care is in fact a human right for all people.

THE TRADITION OF THE COMMON GOOD

Before I began the section on human rights and health care, I mentioned that the topic of health care as a right would need to be grounded in two key themes from the Catholic moral tradition, the common good and the meaning of justice. The Catholic tradition's teaching on the common good is rooted in the works of Aristotle and Aquinas. In our times an understanding of the common good is especially important for U.S. society with its strong tendency toward individualism. The fundamental definition of the common good is that there exists a good for society as a whole which respects but is ultimately more important than the good of any individual.[21] Earlier, when speaking about the natural law tradition, we emphasized natural law's belief in the possibility of good government and good society. It was these themes which generated the strong role of the common good in Catholic thought. Today, in the context of health care reform, it may be that an awareness of which health services most truly foster the common good will be able to stand as a basis for some of the difficult policy decisions which will have to be made as part of health care reform.

Two important cautions are necessary in speaking about the common good. First, we cannot limit our notion of the common good to a focus on material goods alone. The great neo-Thomist Jacques Maritain pointed out in the 1940s that the spiritual good of the individual person transcends the common material good of society.[22] Thus a notion of the common good which denies the existence of God and the spiritual nature of human life is unacceptable, as is any rationale which concentrates on economic productivity to the exclusion of other values. Maritain's concern about Marxist notions of community is obvious, but it also seems that he would be critical of themes such as the famous statement that what is good for General Motors is good for the country. Pope John Paul II's 1991 encyclical *Centesimus Annus* raises a concern very similar to Maritain's when the holy father asserts that socialism's error is that it considers the individual person simply as a molecule within the social organism so that the good of the individual is completely subordinated to the socio-economic mechanism.[23]

In response to Maritain's concerns, what we need is a wholistic notion of the common good which considers all facets of who we are as human persons. For instance, how much will a new health care system give all people a true sense of participation and partnership in the direction of their health care? How much will a new health care system enhance the quality of life and the character of relationships between persons? Will a new health care system foster values like realism about our human limits, peace-making, care for the environment, acceptance of the meaning of death, etc.? These questions are not easy, but if we only ask the more material questions (how much will a new system cost? what number of people can it help?) we will not be working from a sufficiently human grasp of the common good.

The second caution about the common good is that we should not think that the common good relates only to matters of law and public policy. Catholic scholarship makes a distinction between the common good and the public order.[24] The public order refers to that aspect of the common good which is appropriately dealt with through laws and government actions. But the common good itself is a larger notion. Institutions such as hospitals, universities, and drug companies can and should be working for the common good. So should private individuals. In the end, the best system of health care will probably come about through a number of different individuals and groups working together with government for the good.

When I was a young student of theology, the common good was a very frequent theme in Catholic thought. I first learned the term in Latin, since it was such a standard part of Catholic thinking about law and public policy. Thus while I was doing research for this book, I was rather surprised to find that since Vatican II relatively little has been written in Catholic circles about the common good.[25] In the past few years, the University of Notre Dame has sponsored some important new work on the common good, but before that there was almost nothing for a twenty year period.

Charles Curran suggests several reasons why Catholic philosophers and theologians have shown little recent interest in the common good.[26] The teachings of the popes have not stressed the common good as much as in the past. The natural law tradition, on which the concept of the common good rests, is still important but not as central in Catholic moral theology as it once was, now that we are emphasizing things like scripture as sources of moral wisdom. The static, somewhat a-historical view of society in which earlier common good thinking was rooted has been replaced by a more dynamic and historical understanding, an understanding attentive to the signs of the times. The scholar Dennis McCann thinks that the change to a more historical worldview means that we should avoid the traditional notion of the common good, although McCann does suggest a similar but clearly more dynamic and processive phrase, "the good to be pursued in common."[27]

Curran wrote his comments about the decline of Catholic writing about the common good before the publication of Pope John Paul II's *Centesimus Annus* which does bemoan the growing inability—even in the democracies—to situate particular interests within a coherent vi-

sion of the common good.[28] So it may be that the common good theme
will make a comeback in Catholic thought, and in Protestant thought
as well.[29] I think that Curran is generally correct in his summary of
reasons for the decline of interest in the common good. But in addition to Curran's list of reasons, I also think that there may be another
factor, namely that some Catholic thinkers—like so many others in
our society—may have unconsciously adopted many of the individualistic assumptions which mark present day life in the U.S. At this time
in our history we may well need more accurate and carefully nuanced
terms instead of the traditional term "common good." But whatever
the terms, I think it is critically necessary for us to recover the heart of
the common good tradition, for health care reform and for a whole
host of other issues as well.

One of the most fascinating contemporary efforts to restore something of the common good tradition can be found in the book *The
Good Society*,[30] written by Robert Bellah and those who were his co-
authors in the earlier book *Habits of the Heart*.[31] While Bellah and his
groups are working principally as sociologists, it is remarkable how
many theological resources they draw upon, including authors like
the two Niebuhrs and John Courtney Murray, as well as the Catholic
social encyclicals. The title of their book *The Good Society*, borrowed
from a 1937 work by Walter Lippmann, is deliberately chosen in
distinction from the possible title "The Great Society." I think the title
they choose avoids generating any kind of false optimism about what
we can accomplish and instead helps us think more about the quality
of the community which it is possible for us to have together.

The Good Society focuses in particular on social institutions such as
the economic establishment, the government, structures to provide
education, and the churches. The decision to call the book "The Good
Society" instead of "The Good Community" flows precisely from the
authors' intention to highlight the importance of structures, rather
than trusting all community building efforts in the realm of personal
relationships.[32] *The Good Society* affirms the value of government, education, church, etc., and stresses the role of these institutions in helping break down the individualism which marks so much of today's life.
While the background of *The Good Society* is somewhat different, it is
hard not to feel a strong sense of continuity between the book's main
premise and the arguments offered by Aristotle and Aquinas centuries ago.

Of special importance are some of the qualities which the Bellah
group thinks are essential for the working of the good society. They
mention themes such as attentiveness, generativity, responsibility,

trust, and sustainability.[33] To me, all these themes re-echo the concern that the common good not be limited to what is economically or numerically most efficient, but that rather the pursuit of the common good serve to create a society in which all people have a genuine sense of participation rather than alienation.

In the area of health care, I realize that common good judgments will need to ask some of the hard questions which seem to have more quantifiable answers. How much will it cost to develop and/or provide such a technology? How many or how few people will the technology benefit? What sort of benefit does a given technology bring? Does a technology actually save lives, or does it have the worthwhile objective of helping chronic but not life threatening conditions? Will the technology benefit a group such as children who may gain a very long lifespan through the use of the technology? Or will it benefit persons whose earthly lives, even under the best conditions, will end within a few years anyway? These are fair questions, and it is reasonable to consider them.

What the common good tradition shows us, however, is that for true health care reform we must be willing to move beyond the quantifiable questions and move toward a more complete vision of the meaning of human life, toward a vision in which issues like participation, attentiveness, and creativity are an inherent part of the decision making process. If society can recapture a sense of these latter issues, the quantifiable issues can be approached with true justice, so that genuine health care reform becomes a possibility. Without the presence of these broader common good issues, my judgment is that an "every person for himself or herself" outlook about health care will continue to predominate so that real health care reform will be difficult if not impossible.

JUSTICE AND HEALTH CARE

Justice is a crucial moral notion for us to reflect upon in the context of health care reform, a notion which can help us ground human rights including the right to an adequate level of health care. Justice can also help us move beyond the individualist orientation which can mark some rights thinking. In classic Catholic thought justice is understood as a virtue, as one of those stable ongoing habits which mark all aspects of human relationships. The object or purpose of the virtue of justice is that we give each person his or her due, give each person those goods and services which he or she rightfully expects from us. Even from this basic definition it can be seen that justice shifts our thinking from what we can claim from each other to what we *owe* to each other. In other words, justice is about duties and responsibilities, about building the good community. Justice is not simply a question of what we might like to do for other people, not a question of how we might be generous to others. Rather it is a question of what we simply must do for others on the basis of our common humanity. This is not to say that voluntary charitable efforts to better society are unimportant. But such efforts are not enough. They do not meet the demands of justice.

This section on justice will have four parts: first, an outline of the classic Catholic concepts of justice; second, a review of some of the more recent concepts of justice; third, some summary comments on the centrality of distributive justice; fourth, a reflection on which specific principle or canon of justice ought to apply in terms of supplying people with access to health care.

The Classic Catholic Teaching on Justice

COMMUTATIVE JUSTICE

Historically, Roman Catholicism has spoken about three aspects of the claim which justice makes upon us, three types of justice.[34] The first of these, commutative justice, is perhaps the easiest to understand. Commutative justice describes the obligations which exist between two individual people, the obligations which one specific person owes to another person. For instance, if I agree to pay someone $40 to dig a certain size ditch and he digs the ditch exactly to my specifications, I must in commutative justice pay him the $40. If it were a hot day and he did the job very quickly and well, I might also be generous and give him a cold beer, but I must in justice give him the $40.

Commutative justice brings to mind previously set contracts, but there can be other commutative justice relationships as well. The individual employer surely has an obligation to provide just wages, even when economic conditions shift so as to make a previous agreement about wages inadequate. In general, commutative justice is not the major focus in the larger social issue of health care reform since we are speaking about the need for a global system of health care reform, rather than about relationships between specific individuals. However, there are aspects of health care delivery in which commutative justice has a high importance. Consider for instance the relationship between an individual hospital and its nurses, housekeepers, maintenance personnel, etc. Consider also the relationship between the caregivers and specific patients. In relationships such as these, the traditional notion of commutative justice surely applies.[35]

Commutative justice is also important because it can serve as a paradigm for some of the larger notions of justice which we are about to consider. At the level of imagination, it can be hard to develop a vision of what we as a country owe to our citizens in terms of health care. The issue can seem too big to get a hold on. If we can think of the U.S. as a person relating to each one of us as persons, possibly we can begin to activate our creative imaginations about the justice issues. In this context it is interesting to recall that the word "corporation" originally applied to governments as well as to businesses, and that part of the idea behind corporation was that both governments and businesses should be understood as corporate persons having clear public responsibilities to other persons.[36]

LEGAL JUSTICE

The second traditional notion of justice is legal justice, sometimes called general justice. This type of justice has to do with what we as individuals owe to the community. If, as Aristotle and Thomas argued, the community was created and exists for our good, then surely we as individuals are responsible for providing the community with the means which it needs to serve the good of all of us. The requirement of military service is seen by many as an example of legal justice, even though there are continuing debates about pacifism and the nature of just wars.[37] Taxes are another example of legal justice. We can debate the specifics of tax policy, but even in an era when taxes are unpopular, the principle of some taxation so that government can serve the good is unquestionable in the judgment of most people. Still another example of legal justice is the requirement that everyone take appropriate care of the environment. In general, legal justice is very much dependent on the theme of the common good which we considered in the last section of this chapter.

Legal or general justice has important implications in the area of health care. If we agree that an adequate level of health care is a human right, then the citizenry clearly has an obligation to supply society with the goods which it needs to assure that all people in fact have access to adequate health care. This supplying of society with the goods it needs to accomplish health care can take place in various ways, ways which involve both private and public systems of health care delivery. Inevitably, in differing historical circumstances there will be changes in just what goods society needs to deliver health care as well as changes in the means which society uses to assure health care delivery. My view is that today the United States needs a more active government role in assuring access to health care, so that the obligation of legal justice will center more strongly on the obligation of citizens to supply government (not simply society in general) with the ability to assure adequate access to health care.

I am sure it is clear that we cannot address the exact specifics of what we owe society and government as a matter of legal justice in the area of health care, unless we are clear as to the exact specifics of what society and government ought to supply all people in the area of health care. No doubt many of the current frustrations about tax policy in the U.S. come from uncertainty as to how tax monies will be spent and from uncertainty about whether the goals of some government programs are truly reasonable and just. This is true in health care and in many other areas. Thus we cannot speak effectively about legal justice without also considering the third of the traditional Catholic concepts of justice, the concept of distributive justice.

DISTRIBUTIVE JUSTICE

Distributive justice is the obligation which falls on society as a whole in relationship to individual persons. Based on distributive justice, society must meet the reasonable claims of its citizens. As with the other types of justice, distributive justice can be executed differently in different historical settings and with respect to different specific issues. Both private social entities and governments can be involved in the effort to meet the claims of distributive justice. In my view, distributive justice is the most crucial and central of all the justice questions, especially in health care, and especially for the purposes of this book. In the first part of this chapter, we argued that a basic standard of care is a human right for all people. This immediately raises the question of society's responsibility for health care, i.e. the question of distributive justice. Unless we can come up with an adequate understanding of just what society owes to its people in the area of health care, all our other questions about just health care delivery become quite empty.

As a Catholic thinking about distributive justice, it is impossible not to reflect on the pioneering work of the social activist priest, Msgr. John A. Ryan, a moral theologian who did so much to turn Catholic America's attention toward the issues of justice and rights. His classic book, *Distributive Justice,* first published in 1916, stands as a major treatise on the make-up of human community and on the responsibility of the community to share its benefits with all those who are part of the community.[38] With particular emphasis on the field of economics,

Ryan wrote about the four sources which contribute to the worth of any product: the providers of the raw materials from which the product is made, the providers of the capital to develop the raw materials, the managers who oversee the production of the product, and the laborers who make the product. Ryan insisted that each of these groups, especially the laborers, must be justly compensated in a measure which respects the radical human dignity of all. He searched probingly for canons or principles on which the distribution of justice should be based.[39] Clearly much in Ryan's work is dated today, but his central thesis on distributive justice remains crucially important, as does his confidence in the feasibility of a mixed economy, i.e. an economy which retains private enterprise, but with enough social controls to ensure true justice. Ryan died in 1945, long before today's health care crisis, but there is little doubt that his methodology would cause him to be a major advocate of health care reform if he were on the scene for today's debates about health care.

These comments on distributive justice conclude our summary of the traditional threefold Catholic approach to justice. We will return to the precise question of a canon or norm for distributing health care, but we first need to consider two other notions of justice which are prominent today.

Two Modern Notions of Justice

EGALITARIAN JUSTICE

Much of the contemporary discussion about justice focuses on the radical equality of all human beings, leading some authors to speak about egalitarian justice, a term which echoes the famous *liberté, égalité, fraternité* slogan of the French revolution and the "all men are created equal" language of the U.S. Declaration of Independence. It is true that all human persons are radically equal and that any sound theory of justice must respect this fact. There are, however, certain philosophical problems about the egalitarian notion of justice. While we are all equal as humans, we do as individuals have different abilities and talents, all of which can work together for the building of the human community. It may well be just for society, acting for the sake of the whole, to give individuals opportunities to develop their differing gifts, even if this means that not every individual is treated in exactly the same way. Similarly, as individuals we can bear different kinds of burdens, especially in an area like health. Some persons with chronic diseases, physical handicaps, developmental disabilities, and other complicated health conditions may very reasonably expect a level of support from the community which other persons should not expect.[40] In addition, there is the whole question of the preferential option for the poor as well as other types of affirmative action programs in which something other than equal treatment seems to be the most just.[41] For all these reasons, I believe that the distribution question—how society allocates benefits and burdens through the entire community—is ultimately more central to justice than the equality question, even though equality remains hugely important. In this I agree with what Charles E. Curran has written in another context.[42]

SOCIAL JUSTICE

Another concept of justice which occurs a great deal in contemporary thought is the concept of social justice. Today many people use the term social justice in a broad general sense to cover any justice issue which relates to society as a whole. However in its origin in Catholic thought, especially under Pope Pius XI, social justice referred specifically to institutions (governments, corporations, international trade structures, etc.) and to the impact which these institutions can have on the just quality of life for all peoples.[43] Such a notion of social justice has opened the way to a significant critique of institutions and to a significant challenge to institutions to be more just. To the extent that modern health care facilities are institutions and are part of today's economic system with its concern about the "bottom line," the critiques from the Catholic approach to social justice ought to be applied to them. But here again, reform of the structures of society so that society can more effectively deliver health care still depends on society's having a clearer focus on just what health care goods it ought to be delivering to people. Thus, while the social structures question, like the equality question, is a pivotal aspect of all justice including health care justice, my judgment is that the distribution question (i.e. What health care benefits must we provide?) is the most central of all the justice questions which relate to health care.

Some Summary Comments on Distributive Justice

At the beginning of this book I stated that the concept of distributive justice would be the most synthetic of all the moral notions addressed in the book. Just now, in describing five categories or types of justice, I have again indicated the centrality of distributive justice. In many respects, the case for distributive justice can stand quite well on its own merits. It simply makes the most sense to begin by asking what it is we must do for all people in terms of supplying them with access to health care. How can we say anything else about justice in the delivery of health care, unless we conceive of society as having responsibilities to its citizens, and unless we see reasonable access to health care as one of these social responsibilities? If we do feel a sense of moral outrage about the thirty-seven million uninsured persons in the U.S., is not the outrage due to our country's failure to meet the demands of distributive justice? As noted earlier, these comments do not resolve the issues of exactly how health care should be distributed, or exactly what level of health care should be supplied. But there is no doubt that the fundamental claim is a claim of distributive justice.

It is also helpful to note that each of the other categories of justice, while valid and important, falls well short of establishing a sufficiently wholistic basis for approaching the question of justice and health care. If we focus too strongly on commutative justice, we are too likely to understand health care in terms of a market economy, with all the problems noted earlier about an overly market-oriented approach to health care.[44] If we focus too much on legal justice, we are very likely to get so preoccupied with the tax burdens involved in just health care that we fail to focus on the core issue of what we owe one another with regard to health care. It is true that there are complex questions about how to levy taxes and about the need to build an economy which is productive enough to sustain just tax burdens in an area such as health care. But these are not the most pivotal questions about health care justice.

If we focus too much on egalitarian notions of justice, we may become overly concerned about how to justify affirmative action for health and about access for some persons to health care services which go beyond the minimum which we must supply to all. If we focus too much on social justice, the risk is that we will emphasize the structures necessary to furnish health care instead of first focusing on the human need of real persons to have real health care crises adequately addressed. Such emphasis on structures without a prior commitment to genuine human needs can raise all the fears of complex bureaucracies without really substantial goals. Once we consider all these limits of the other categories, the case for distributive justice as the central notion of health care justice becomes even clearer.

Toward a Canon of Distributive Justice for Health Care Delivery

If distributive justice is so central to health care reform, we need to come up with some kind of canon or principle for distributive justice in health care. In general, apart from health care, theologians and philosophers engage in an ongoing effort to come up with a suitable norm or theory of distributive justice. One well-known modern effort at a norm for justice can be found in John Rawls' *A Theory of Justice*, published in 1971.[45] Rawls argues that distribution of benefits in a society must be equal for all except when it can be shown that giving more benefits to some people enables those who have less to have more than they would have had otherwise. Thus if a policy which makes rich people richer serves to make the poor less poor it is a just policy. Many criticisms are made of Rawls, both in terms of whether his theory actually works, and in terms of whether the poor, even if they have a little more materially, are not even more alienated personally under Rawls' approach so that the overall human condition of society is actually worsened.

In terms of the specific question of distributive justice in health care, my view is that the work of the Protestant theologian Gene Outka in the mid-1970s is the most significant single contribution to the modern effort to work out a theory of distributive justice for the health care field.[46] Later we will be talking about the work of Daniel Callahan (with his notion of limits) and about the Catholic Health Association's working group on rationing.[47] To me it seems that these very notable efforts all have roots in Outka's notion of distributive justice.

Outka considers five possible canons or maxims of distributive justice for health care. First is the distribution of health care benefits based on people's merit. Such a meritarian approach to justice ignores the fact that health care needs can occur completely independently of merit. In addition how can we humans, with our weaknesses and biases, really assess the merit or virtue of one person against another? There may be a few narrow cases where meritarian notions could be used in health care distribution, such as giving non-smokers slightly lower insurance rates. But on the whole, merit is surely an inadequate canon for distributing health care justly.

Outka's second possible canon is the distribution of health care benefits to persons based on their social usefulness, i.e. the more useful persons are, the better health care they get. Here again, health care needs can be very much disconnected from social usefulness, especially when we consider that health care needs tend to be particularly prominent in children and even more so in older persons. Also, how can we really tell who is more useful? Do we understand enough about the human good to make such a judgment? In this context it is hard not to think about Paul Ramsey's account of the early efforts of the Swedish Hospital in Seattle to decide who should get kidney dialysis. Noting that the hospital committee which made these decisions tended to pick out persons whose social status was much like their own, Ramsey ended up by quoting the famous remark that the Pacific Northwest would be a very bad place in which to be a Henry David Thoreau with bad kidneys.[48]

There may be some very rare circumstances in which the focus of all society or of a specific social group is clear enough that health care benefits might be distributed to the society or the group on the basis of social worth. One thinks for instance of battlefield triage which aims to quickly attend to those who can continue the fight so that even more people will not end up being killed, captured or wounded by the enemy. Another example, not directly connected to health care, comes from the famous Holmes case in which it was decided that after a ship sank in the North Atlantic, at least some sailors had to be saved to handle the lifeboats, or in the end no one would be saved. In the end, I think the very character of these exceptions shows that in ordinary circumstances we cannot use social worth as a principle for the just distribution of health care.

Outka's third possible canon of distribution is a system of providing people with health care based on their ability to pay for it. Outka argued against this position in 1974, noting particularly that in view of the overall human importance of health care crises, it seems out of place to force people to consider how much they can afford to pay for their health care.[49] Outka took his position on this issue before the crisis in U.S. health care delivery reached the proportions which we are aware of today. If anything, his arguments against the ability to pay as the principle for delivering health care are even clearer than when he first proposed them.

In saying this, I would not deny that there may be certain health care services which go beyond the basic needed minimum and that these services might be made available on the basis of ability to pay. But this would only be true if the assured minimum were clearly adequate and in place for all people. Also, not every conceivable service beyond the basic package should be available to those who can pay. If a proposed service involved an undue risk, or drained away resources needed for other goods, I think society could bar such a health care service, even from those who could pay for it on an optional basis.

After having dealt with merit, usefulness, and economic ability, Outka turns to the two canons of just health care delivery which he thinks have the highest potential for turning out to be correct. The first of these (fourth overall) rests in the famous maxim "To each according to his needs." Even though this maxim has a Marxist tone, it immediately strikes us as attractive. After all health care is about sick and therefore needy people. Meeting these needs seems to be a basic goal. Once we get rid of the false notions found in the first three canons, why should we not make the meeting of health care needs our basic canon for the just distribution of health care services?

Surely the human need for health care must always be part of our consciousness when we seek to develop a just system of health care. We should always want to do whatever we can to meet people's legitimate health care needs. Thus the canon "To each according to her needs" stands as an energy behind our approach to health care and as at least a partial answer in the quest for justice. It must always be part of our thinking about health care justice.

But can the canon based on need be the final answer? Once we grant some of the facts we discussed earlier, i.e. that sickness and death are inevitable, we realize that as finite human beings it will not be possible for us to make available every conceivable service in the area of health care. This leads Outka to his fifth and ultimately most correct canon of health care justice which is "similar treatment for similar cases."[50] In other words, with careful reflection and dialogue, we should determine those health care needs which we as a society must meet as a minimum standard, and then provide these needs for everyone, regardless of merit, usefulness, economic ability, etc. Such an approach means that there will be some possible health services which will not be provided because they are not truly needs or because they are beyond our capacity as a society of mortals who must face the fact of death. To use Callahan's phrase, similar treatment for similar cases will involve us in setting limits.[51]

It is interesting to consider how classic Catholic thought relates to this theme of establishing a decent minimum standard for health care and then assuring that everyone has access to the minimum standard. In classic Catholic thought about the living wage, it was assumed that if all persons could live in reasonable and frugal comfort, their true needs (as opposed to wants) were being met and that distributive justice was being achieved. Classic Catholic thought held that our understanding of the nature and dignity of the human person was such that we could know which goods and services were necessary for a person to live in reasonable and frugal comfort.

In health care, if we decide that the development of one life-extending technology will deny us the opportunity to develop another life-extending technology which has even more potential to extend lives, it may well be that persons who are hoping for the first technology will assert that they are being denied a true health care need. If we accept the fact that death is intrinsic to human existence and that the goodness of life is an instrumental good, it can be argued that the extension of life is not always an absolute need, especially if the common good ultimately outranks the individual good. Such an approach would make the "similar treatment/minimum standard" approach to health care justice very close to classic Catholic thought, but the tension remains around the issue of not developing every possible life-extending technology. Clearly, the theology of death which we reviewed in Chapter 3 has a crucial importance in the debate about distributive justice and health care. We can only hope to focus a minimum standard of care which society must provide to everyone after we have accepted the idea that death is a part of life.

We will consider many of these issues further in a section about health care rationing, but for now the point is that the canon about setting a basic minimum standard of similar treatment for similar cases stands as the best approach to distributive justice in health care. As soon as we say this, the matter of legal justice also comes to the fore, i.e. the responsibility of all of us (through taxes, other funding mechanisms, and creative private health services) to be sure that society has the resources it needs to provide a basic set of health care services to all people.

In contexts other than health care some scholars have raised questions about the theme of disinterested love which underlies Outka's appeal to the theme of similar treatment for similar cases. It is argued for instance that we owe more to our parents than we do to other people.[52] I agree that in some kinds of situations we do owe more to some people than to others. But in terms of a nation setting a policy on how to deliver health care justly, it is clear that the setting up of a basic standard of similar treatment for similar cases makes the most sense. The one area in which we might wonder about the adequacy of the similar treatment for similar cases approach has to do with the poor and other groups in society about whom it is said that we should make a preferential option. My view is that the option for the poor involves a requirement that we take the necessary procedural steps to be sure that the poor, cultural minorities, etc., are fully aware that they have access to just health care as a matter of right. However, the actual level of health care services to be made available to the poor need not be different from what we provide to everyone else.

WHAT ABOUT HEALTH CARE RATIONING?

In our survey of current developments and proposals in Chapter 2, we mentioned some of the pros and cons of the Oregon plan of health care rationing. Now, in light of all the ethical reflection of the past few chapters, it is time to inquire more directly about whether health care rationing can ever be a moral option. For the purposes of our inquiry, health care rationing can be defined as the decision not to develop or not to provide people with potentially beneficial medical treatments.

As a moral theologian, my view is that health care rationing can in fact be justifiable. As soon as we consider that we are finite human beings and that, as a matter of both philosophy and faith, death is inevitable, it becomes clear that in the nature of things there are limits as to how much we should and ought to do to prolong life and to prevent death. In some historical eras such as ours, it may seem necessary for the sake of the common good to use public policy to help us recognize the natural limits of life in the first place. No ultimate moral objection need be lodged against such a use of public policy, even if there is a need for careful moral scrutiny of any specific rationing plan.

In asserting the moral possibility of health care rationing, it is hard not to think about how health care relates to other crucial common good issues such as education. To put it simply, if we spend every conceivable dollar to develop and furnish potentially beneficial health care services, we will take so much money away from education that we could very quickly become a nation of illiterates (a tragedy which is already happening in some places).[53] In another generation, it might happen that no one will have the educational abilities to use all of our wonderful medical technologies. If so, then the last situation would be worse than the first.

In Chapter 1, I mentioned that by the very fact of the many millions of uninsured persons in our country, the United States already has a health care rationing plan in effect. The current plan works against the poor, against those who work for small employers, and against some racial and ethnic minorities. It is clearly an unjust approach to rationing because similar health care needs are not treated in a similar way for all persons and there is no assured basic level of access to health care. In the real world, therefore, the question is not whether or not we ought to have health care rationing. The real question is how to come up with an appropriately just plan of health care rationing.

My own position is to argue that the rationing of potentially beneficial health care services can be justified under the following seven conditions. First, a move toward rationing of health care services must be a last resort, i.e. all other efforts to deliver a reasonable level of health care must be tried and found to fall short of the goals of a just health care policy. More efficient approaches to delivery, alternative delivery settings, etc., must all be employed to their maximum potential before rationing is considered. Our review of these prior steps earlier in the book has suggested that they are not sufficient, so that rationing is in fact justifiable. In stating this last-resort condition, it seems as though I am making the case for rationing sound similar to the case for a just war. But due to the enormous moral importance of just health care delivery, it may not be inappropriate to use language which makes us think about an issue as sobering as war.

Second, before it begins any program of health care rationing, our society needs to develop a clear consensus on the question of medical futility, using the kind of principles I outlined in Chapter 4. Based on this clear consensus, patients as a matter of medical policy should not be provided with any futile treatments. It seems unconscionable for us to speak about withholding beneficial treatments if at the same time we are continuing to furnish some people with futile treatments. Obviously there are questions about framing the concept of futility correctly, and about leaving patients with appropriate discretion in borderline cases. But addressing the futility question is an essential preliminary to any just rationing program.

Third, a program of health care rationing must be set up so that in the long run it requires involvement in the program by all members of U.S. society, not just involvement by some groups within a society such as the poor. To be effective, a rationing program designed for the whole of society must furnish a high enough standard of care that most people are quite satisfied to participate in the program and accept what it provides.[54] It must be clear that the rationing program does a good job in meeting people's essential health care needs. Otherwise there would be constant complaints about the program, and a general level of instability.

The assertion that a health care rationing program must be designed so as to require involvement by all people does not mean that we can do without a special concern about the health care needs of the poor. Especially as a health care rationing program is starting up, there will need to be an emphasis on the poor because of all the health care they have lacked in the past. But to be fully just, a rationing program must be designed for society as a whole so that it is taken for granted that the poor have access to the same basic package of services which is available to everyone else. This is what the fundamental notion of human dignity requires of us. To my way of thinking, this is the point of Outka's "similar treatment for similar cases" criterion, i.e. that a basic level of services must be made available to all persons.

Fourth, a program whose focus on human dignity provides a decent or reasonable level of rationed care to every citizen need not exclude all seeking of additional optional health related services by those who can pay for them. However, if any type of optional access to health care becomes so consumptive of health care resources that it threatens basic access to health care services or threatens our ability to provide other social goods such as education, housing, or defense, this type of optional health care ought to be excluded.

Fifth, while a just program of health care rationing must be aware of the needs of every individual person, its ultimate focus must be on the common good in the wholistic sense of common good which I described earlier. Among the many common good issues which must be part of any just rationing program, I would especially stress two issues: participation and non-discrimination. In terms of participation, decisions on how to ration health care services should be made on the basis of dialogue with as large a segment of the human community as possible. Health care professionals, economists, political leaders, religious leaders, philosophers and theologians, business and labor leaders, media representatives, and spokespersons for public interest groups should all be part of the dialogue. Persons with different kinds of diseases should have a special chance to be part of the dialogue and to state their needs. Also it is crucially necessary that advocates for the poor be part of the dialogue process in working out any plan for health care rationing.

In terms of non-discrimination, the common good requires that factors such as religion, race, economic status, and talent ought never to be the basis for deciding who is eligible for what in a basic package of health care services. If we discriminated for these reasons, how could we be said to have a health care policy which is committed to the common good?

Gender works a little differently as a discrimination factor since there can be kinds of medical services which members of one or the other sex need precisely because of their differing physiology. For these kinds of services the standard should be that the needed service be available to all members of the pertinent sex regardless of any other factors. Beyond these specifically sexually related services, there should be no difference in basic services because of one's sex.

Age is also a tricky factor in terms of the common good and health care delivery. I think there can be no discrimination in excluding age-appropriate medical services from any person from the infant to the centenarian. But I also think there is room for reasonable debate on just which services are appropriate for persons in given age brackets. Very complex surgeries, with lengthy recovery periods and only limited prospects for success, may sometimes be appropriate for young persons but not for persons whose age is quite advanced. Other countries have worked out policies on such issues, and the U.S. might do well to see what it can learn from the experience of such countries.

Sixth, a rationing policy can only be just in withholding a potentially beneficial medical treatment when the burden connected with that treatment is a burden which is found in the treatment itself, rather than a burden based on a societal judgment that the life of the person from whom the treatment is withheld would be too burdensome even if the treatment were provided. If a treatment is very costly (a classic issue in Catholic medical ethics), is hard to acquire, has uncertain results, or threatens our ability to provide more basic services, society may have a reasonable case for choosing not to provide such a treatment. But if it is not too difficult for society to provide the treatment, and if the treatment itself does not cause the patient undue burden, I do not believe there is a ground for a social policy which excludes such a treatment. Earlier we argued that a patient or those entitled to speak for him or her might refuse non-burdensome treatment because the treatment will result in a burdensome life. My point now is that to respect patient autonomy, these kinds of delicate borderline decisions ought to be left in the hands of patients rather than becoming part of a rationing policy. This does not mean that patients can demand futile treatments or treatments which can only be furnished with great prejudice to the common good. But I do think it is important to preserve a zone of patient autonomy in addressing some of these very delicate issues.

Seventh, because medicine and socio-economic conditions change so rapidly, a health care rationing policy can only be just if it undergoes frequent periodic review to be sure that it is providing the maximum level of effective services. This review ought to include the same kind of broad dialogue which the development of a rationing policy should involve in the first place.

Among the growing array of very useful resource materials on the rationing question, I find Daniel Callahan's *What Kind of Life? The Limits of Medical Progress* to be the most helpful contribution.[55] Also very helpful is the Catholic Health Association (CHA)'s pamphlet *With*

Justice For All? The Ethics of Health Care Rationing which was prepared by a group of distinguished scholars.[56] Like my own summary above, the CHA pamphlet lists a set of criteria for health care rationing. Our two lists are quite similar but not exactly the same. In my summary, besides many of the issues addressed by the CHA group, I have tried to show how issues like medical futility, burdensome quality of life, and optional treatments might relate to a rationing program.

HEALTH CARE REFORM: GOVERNMENT INVOLVEMENT VS. PRIVATE INITIATIVE

The final social/moral issue for our consideration in this chapter has to do with a theme we have mentioned several times, namely that there seems to be an important place in health care delivery for both private initiative and government involvement. But how do we balance the private and the governmental aspects of health care delivery? Is there any Catholic social teaching which can add to our perspective on this issue? To answer we need to consider the well-known discussion of subsidiarity and socialization which has occurred in the papal social encyclicals of the twentieth century.

One of the most interesting parts of Pope Pius XI's 1931 encyclical *Quadragesimo Anno* was the holy father's discussion of the principle of subsidiarity.[57] According to this principle, things which can be handled effectively by private initiative ought to be handled that way. Similarly, matters which can be handled effectively by a lower level of government (i.e. a city government instead of a state government, a state government instead of a national government) ought to be handled by the lower government. The role of the higher levels of government is to provide help (this is the meaning of the word "subsidy" from which the principle of subsidiarity takes its name) for those matters which the lower groups cannot handle by themselves. The end result of the principle of subsidiarity is that there will be a healthy pluralism of approaches present as society seeks to address various social problems.[58]

Historically it is clear that Pius XI was making a greater opening to government involvement in social and economic issues. But he wanted to do this very cautiously, and thus generated the idea of subsidiarity which makes it clear that only that level of government involvement which is truly necessary ought to take place. Pius XI's ghostwriter for *Quadragesimo Anno*, the Jesuit Oswald von Nell-Bruening, lived to be more than one hundred and died only in 1991, so that even in recent years Catholic scholars have been able to have a pipeline into the thought world of *Quadragesimo Anno.*

None of the popes since Pius XI have disputed the principle of subsidiarity. Beginning, however, with Pope John XXIII's encyclical *Mater et Magistra,* there has been a tendency for the popes to say that the world is growing ever more complex and that therefore more government involvement is in fact necessary to meet the demands of social justice. In *Mater et Magistra,* John XXIII summed up this line of thinking with the famous term "socialization," a term repeated in a similar context by Pope John Paul II in *Laborem Exercens.*[59] Since the publication of *Mater et Magistra,* many Catholic thinkers have used the two terms "subsidiarity" and "socialization" to describe the tension between private or local government initiatives and the social programs of state or national governments. In the decades after *Mater et Magistra,* several of the social encyclicals have had a "north-south" focus (stressing relations between the developed and the underdeveloped countries) while other encyclicals have had more of an "east-west" focus (stressing relations between capitalism and communism). Especially in the north-south encyclicals (such as *Populorum Progressio* and *Sollicitudo Rei Socialis*) there has been a continuing emphasis on John XXIII's theme of the need for more government activities to help bring about a more just world.

It should be no surprise that some conservative Roman Catholics have not been happy with John XXIII's emphasis on socialization and with some of the other more recent social teaching. William F. Buckley's famous phrase "mater, si, magistra, no" sums up much of this conservative critique. Sometimes, also, this conservative critique will interpret the social encyclicals as having a stronger pro-capitalist tone than is actually the case.[60] It is important that we not twist the careful balance of Catholic teaching toward socialism. But at the same time we should not underemphasize the place of socialization in Catholic social teaching.

In terms of health care, the Catholic social teaching on subsidiarity/socialization can tell us two important things. First, we really do need to find a health care system which offers us some balance between private management and public management. In this context it will remain very hard to justify something like the British system in which the public sector has such a dominant role in both access and delivery. Second, in view of the increasingly complex character of health care delivery, it is only to be expected (and clearly "catholic") that more and more government management of health care will in fact be necessary. Thus we ought not to be afraid on religious/moral grounds of the fact that many of the major health care reform proposals which are being discussed in the United States today are calling for a significantly increased level of government involvement, at least in the financing of health care. In the end, Catholic social teaching may well help us decide which of the current reform proposals seem best, by challenging us to consider carefully which proposal best mixes subsidiarity and socialization in our current health care context.

These comments bring us to the end of the second part of this book. In this part we have sought to review the major theological and moral resources which might help us move toward meaningful health care reform. What remains for Part Three will be an effort to assess what that health care reform might look like in practice.

PART THREE

HEALTH CARE REFORM TO COME: THE SHAPE OF THE FUTURE

Chapter 7

THEOLOGY AND THE CHURCHES: THEIR PLACE IN THE HEALTH CARE DEBATE

Part One of this book surveyed the major problems in health care delivery today and reviewed some of the noteworthy proposals for reform. Part Two, working from the viewpoint of Roman Catholicism, explored the resources which theology, ethics, and the churches have to bring to the health care debate. The main task for Part Three will be to try to show just what a reformed health care system might look like in light of the theological and moral perspectives which were presented in Part Two. There is, however, one important preliminary question before we turn to this final task: Just what is the place of the churches and theology in the debate about an issue like health care reform? What do the churches have to say about this matter in comparison with economists, political leaders, health care professionals, etc.? How weighty should the concerns of the churches be in the final shape of a reformed health care system? For the Roman Catholic Church, with its strong emphasis on official moral teaching, how should that official teaching influence the Catholic Church's efforts for health care reform? Chapter 7 will attempt to answer this question, and then Chapter 8, the final chapter, will take up the question of the actual shape of health care reform.

Our answer to the question about the place of theology and the churches in the health care debate will have four main parts. First, we will consider several of the key ecclesiological stances on the matter of religion and public policy, especially the stances of Lutheranism, Calvinism, and Catholicism. Some of the groundwork for looking at these stances was already accomplished in Chapter 5. Second, we will make a more in-depth study of the implications of the Roman Catholic approach to religion and public policy. Third, we will review the traditional Roman Catholic theology of cooperation as it applies to the topic of religion and public policy. Fourth, we will consider some major tension areas in which the Catholic perspective might conflict with the perspectives of economists, politicians, etc. The tension areas we will consider will include the question of a proposed health care system which is lacking in perfect justice, especially in terms of the preferential option for the poor, and the question of a proposed health care system, some of whose provisions are at variance with the Catholic teachings on sexual morality and abortion.

RELIGION AND PUBLIC POLICY: THREE GREAT ECCLESIOLOGICAL TRADITIONS

Earlier, in Chapter 5, we noted that Roman Catholicism has a generally favorable outlook on the potential of civil laws as a means of social reform. But here our question is more specific: To be a good law, how much must a law be in conformity with Catholic moral teaching? Must there be complete conformity? Is there no need for any conformity? Or is there some mediating position between total conformity and complete non-conformity? The Catholic approach to these questions can be best answered if we begin by looking at three distinct ecclesiological positions on the matter of religion and public policy.

Lutheranism

The first position to be considered is the classical Lutheran viewpoint on religion and public policy. In the Lutheran position, there is a sharp and deep gulf between the world of religious morality and the world of public policy. Lutheranism acknowledges that God created the public order. But the public order was created as a result of human sinfulness and it is thoroughly marked by the reality of sin. This means that the state and its laws are to be understood as the "left hand of God," as a "dike against sin." Hence it is completely unrealistic to expect the laws of society to measure up to the moral standards of Christianity. If we try to make our laws measure up to Christian moral standards, the laws will turn out to be worse instead of better. The classic Lutheran position does not object to Christians holding public office. But Christian office holders should not attempt to insert their Christian values into the workings of their political offices. Instead, such Christian officers should make every effort in their private lives to engage in activities which help to make up for some of the questionable results of their activities as office-holders.[1]

Such an ecclesiological stance reduces the effort for health care reform to pure political pragmatism. Even at this level there are still some important energies for health care reform in that our current health care system is having such a negative effect on economic life in the U.S. But in the classic interpretation of Luther's political thought, many of the religious values we have seen in this book—on topics such as justice and human dignity—are not seen as entering into the development of public policies on health care.

It should be noted that the Lutheran perspective does help us by calling us to a sober political realism which can keep us from expecting too much moral perfection in our public policies. If we expect too much of the political process and then fail to get it, we run the risk of giving up altogether on public policy as a means to health care reform. I also want to note that here I have deliberately spoken about the classic Lutheran approach so as to summarize the major aspects of Luther's views on politics, especially as he expressed them in his *Treatise on Secular Authority*.[2] But this classic view should not obscure the fact that many Lutheran thinkers, while retaining Luther's central emphases, have developed approaches to public policy which are more subtle and nuanced.[3]

Calvinism

The second major ecclesiological stance on the relationship between religion and public policy differs dramatically from the Lutheran position. This is the view of John Calvin and those in his tradition. From the Calvinist perspective, for a public policy to be a good public policy it must be in complete accord with Christian moral principles. This stance comes from Calvin's notion that the state is subservient to religious values and should ultimately be controlled by religious leaders. This approach has strength in that it marks politics with an enthusiasm or fervor for the good. Politics becomes dynamic, and it is believed that real political change is possible for the betterment of the human community. The passivity which can sometimes mark the Lutheran approach to politics is dispersed by Calvin's high sense of the union between religion and politics.[4]

But there are also some problems with the Calvinist approach. First, might it not be true that there are some aspects of secular wisdom (in economics, medicine, sociology, etc.) which religion as such is not fully competent to evaluate? If this is so, might it not be better to understand the political process as involving a dialogue between religious morality and sources of secular wisdom, instead of simply construing politics as a tool which religious leadership uses to help educate people into religious moral values? From such a perspective of dialogue, it would seem that religious morality would be especially strong in providing principles to guide the political process, while the various human sciences would be more able to provide insights into specific concrete issues (such as the relative efficiency of various structures for health care financing).

A second potential difficulty with the Calvinist outlook is that since religious leaders are human beings like the rest of us, there may be times when a certain narrowness of vision marks how religious leaders interpret their tradition and apply it to the political process. The history of the U.S. during the Prohibition era is an important example of this kind of situation, and it may well be that the end results of Prohibition were more bad than good, even though there were important moral concerns which led to the establishment of Prohibition.[5] If such a narrowness of vision is occasionally possible, perhaps it would be better to abandon the complete union of religion and politics which Calvin contemplated. Instead of a complete union, there may well be a place for a certain autonomy of politics vis-à-vis religious morality.

Roman Catholicism

These thoughts bring us to the third major ecclesiological vision on religion and politics, i.e. the Roman Catholic position. In the Roman Catholic perspective, as developed by Thomas Aquinas and others, there is no huge gulf between the realm of religious/moral values and the realm of public policy. Instead, public policy is to be acutely conscious of moral issues and it is to strive as far as possible to embody moral standards. Occasionally, one hears a Catholic candidate for political office state something to the effect that "my religion is one thing and my political judgment is a completely separate reality." Such a stance is clearly not the traditional Catholic viewpoint, since in the traditional Catholic outlook the Catholic office holder who has sincere good faith ought to try to imbue his or her politics with genuine moral standards.[6]

At the same time, however, Roman Catholicism realizes that religious morality and political judgment are not completely identical. In addition to its concern for moral standards, politics, which has been traditionally known as the art of the possible, needs to take account of certain aspects of the human condition which may not come within the immediate purview of religious/moral standards.[7] For this reason, sound Christian political judgment may on occasion endorse political initiatives which are not totally in accord with Christian moral stan-

dards. To say this in another way, Catholic moral thought has traditionally recognized the idea that both religious morality and politics ought
to have a certain degree of independence or autonomy in their own
spheres. Some readers may recall that in traditional Catholic teaching
both church and state were said to be "perfect societies."[8] Perfect
societies did not mean that church and state were without flaw. This
term meant rather that both church and state had a certain complete-
ness or ability to operate by themselves. In other words, the tradition
of "perfect societies" was another way in which Catholicism endorsed
the legitimate autonomy of church and of state.

All three of the ecclesiological traditions we have just discussed
make very important contributions to the debate about religion and
public policy. I believe, however, that a good case can be made that the
Catholic approach to religion and politics is the most balanced of the
three major ecclesiological viewpoints which we have just considered.
The Catholic approach avoids both the sharp, pessimistic gulf between religion and public policy and the overly simplistic complete
identification of religion and public policy. In the end, the subtle
Catholic position on this issue is one of the reasons why I am especially
proud to be in the Roman Catholic tradition. Politics always remains a
moral reality, and the challenge to make our politics ever more moral
is constantly present. But at the same time, Catholics can recognize the
legitimate integrity of the political process in and of itself.

SOME SPECIFICS ON THE CATHOLIC APPROACH

Just above I stated that while for Catholics politics must always be a
moral venture, politics may occasionally need to address questions that
will lead it to adopt positions which are not fully in accord with Catholic
moral teaching. What kind of questions are there which might lead
lawmakers to legitimately adopt policies that do not fully embody moral
standards of conduct? These questions, which are often called questions about a law's technical feasibility, fall into a number of different
categories.[9] Here we will consider four of the main technical feasibility
questions.

The first feasibility question has to do with enforceability. Can a
law, even if it has a moral objective, be effectively enforced? If a law is
passed which cannot be enforced, the concern is that the existence of
such an unenforceable law will serve to undermine respect for all laws,
thereby helping to create an unstable and more dangerous society.
Thus it is usually said that it is politically wiser not to pass an unen-

forceable law, even if the law has a solidly moral objective. Much of the discussion about the repeal of the earlier laws which reduced the maximum speed limit in the entire U.S. to fifty-five miles per hour centered on the question of enforceability. Surely, the reduced speed laws had worthy moral purposes: the conservation of energy and the reduction of accidents. No one who favored the repeal of the reduced speed laws questioned the moral goal of these laws. Instead, the arguments for repeal have stated that since laws imposing such a low speed limit are fundamentally unenforceable, it is better not to have such laws with such a low limit in the first place. Similar considerations might well enter into some issues related to health care reform. It probably would not be possible to prevent some health problems (excess weight, smoking related sicknesses) through legislation banning certain types of food intake or the use of tobacco, so in the long run it would be better not to pass such legislation, even if it had a clearly moral objective.

The second question related to the technical feasibility of the law has to do with laws which are intended to be enforced against everyone but which are typically enforced only against certain groups in a society instead of against everyone in the society. Here the standard argument has been that if in concrete fact a law intended for all is only used against certain groups, the law is a bad law, even if it has an ultimate purpose which is moral. An important modern example of this problem of selective enforceability has to do with the issue of capital punishment. In the 1950s, Pope Pius XII taught that there was nothing theoretically wrong with capital punishment from the viewpoint of Catholic moral teaching.[10] But in more recent times the Catholic bishops of the U.S. (and many others) have taken positions opposing capital punishment.[11] The Catholic bishops have made it clear that they are not questioning Pius XII's overall defense of capital punishment. Instead, the Catholic bishops argue that in the U.S. at this time in history it is too likely that capital punishment will be used against persons who are poor or members of racial minorities rather than being used against everyone in society who might commit a capital offense.

This issue of selective enforceability might come to the fore in health care in several ways. For instance, future health care reform legislation might choose to ban the use of certain types of expensive and exotic medical technologies on the ground that the medical resources consumed by these technologies would prevent society from providing a decent level of health care to all persons in the society. If this happens, it would be wrong for society to fail to enforce such a ban against all persons. If the rich were able to find a way around such a law, we would be dealing with selective enforceability.

The third major question on technical feasibility has to do with what kind of law it is actually possible to pass in a society in which there are democratic structures and elected lawmakers who have diverse viewpoints on the nature of moral life. A legislator committed to Catholic moral principles may find that it is possible to pass a law which supports most of his or her moral convictions on a given issue. However it will not be possible to pass a law which embraces all of his or her moral convictions on the issue. If this legislator (and others like him or her) hold out for a law which they find to be one hundred percent moral, the result may be that no law at all will pass and that the public moral climate will be all the worse. In this sort of circumstance, it seems reasonable for a Catholic legislator to support a law which is morally better than existing laws but not perfectly moral. Certainly the Catholic bishops ought to respect the integrity of a legislator's judgment of conscience in this sort of circumstance, even though both the bishops and the legislator may continue to press for still further legislation on the issue at hand. Here we are back to the point that politics is the art of the possible. It is surely reasonable to consider what is possible when evaluating what sort of legislation to support.

This third question about political possibility could well become quite significant if the U.S. Supreme Court should decide that legislation on abortion ought to be a matter left in the hands of the states. If this happens, there could very well be states which would be willing to limit abortions (to cases of rape, incest, etc.), but not to outlaw them altogether. If Catholic legislators in such states were to oppose such laws because they do not completely outlaw abortion, the result could well be that no new laws would be passed and that earlier abortion-on-demand laws would remain in effect. I do not mention this example with a view to resolving all the issues related to abortion and public policy, but I do want to make the point that even with an issue as crucial as abortion, some of the traditional Catholic thinking about morality and public policy may well need to come into play.[12]

The fourth question about the technical feasibility of a law has to do with whether the passage of a law whose basic objectives are clearly moral might for some extrinsic reasons result in more harm than good for society as a whole. This overall greater harm might occur in various ways. The passage of the law might serve to strengthen a political group in the society which has some very dangerous and immoral ultimate objectives such as the starting of an unjust war. The passage of the law might spawn a whole realm of troubling and difficult behaviors. Some argue, for example, that there ought not to be laws against prostitution since these laws would help engender a world of pimps, crime, venereal disease, etc., while failing to prevent prostitution. I am not claiming that I agree with this particular example, but I use it to help show the kind of considerations which can come up when we think about the feasibility of laws in a world which is very much marked by sin and by human finitude.

Other examples of the technical feasibility tradition might also be cited, but I think the main lines of the Roman Catholic tradition on religion and public policy are clear. Roman Catholicism sees itself as called to challenge public policy to be as moral as possible, but it also sees itself as called to respect the total character of the political process with its legitimate autonomy. In reflecting on this, it is hard not to think about Reinhold Niebuhr's warning that in practical life we have to look for proximate solutions to problems, since ultimate solutions may not be achievable and since efforts spent to accomplish ultimate solutions may result in the achievement of nothing at all.[13] No doubt the Roman Catholic tradition will experience tensions and debates about just when it should challenge legislation to be more fully moral and when it ought to accept something less-than-perfect as the most reasonable option in a given set of historical circumstances. In those cases where there are genuinely debatable differences of opinion on such matters, honest differences of opinion between people ought to be respected on the basis of a confidence in the overall soundness of Catholic teaching on religion and public policy.

Cooperation in Evil

The theology of cooperation is another theme in the Roman Catholic moral tradition that can help us to address the issue of public policy on health care which is not in full accord with Catholic moral teaching. As its name suggests, the theology of cooperation raises the issue of when a person or a community might legitimately choose to go along with a practice which the person or community cannot fully support. To understand the theology of cooperation we need to begin by reviewing two key distinctions on cooperation, the distinction between formal and material cooperation, and the distinction between proximate and remote material cooperation.[14]

In formal cooperation, the person supplying the cooperation desires that the evil happen. For instance, if a group of robbers decides to rob a bank, they may appoint one member of the gang to be outside the bank driving the getaway car. Even though the getaway driver does not actually rob the bank, he is clearly part of the evil plot. He offers formal cooperation in the robbery. In material cooperation, the person supplying the cooperation does not desire that the evil happen, but he or she chooses to cooperate in the evil. If the above gang of bank robbers is small, they may all rob the bank and then rush to the street, point a shotgun at the first driver they encounter, and insist that this driver take them to their hideout. In this scenario, the driver of the car may well choose to transport the gang so as not to get his or her head blown off by the shotgun. Here the driver clearly does not intend the evil of the bank robbery. The cooperation is only material cooperation offered under the duress of the situation.

The second distinction is between proximate and remote cooperation. This distinction has to do with the degree of involvement which the cooperator has in the evil of the action. Some cooperation is very closely related to the evil in question, e.g. a nurse preparing a patient for an operation which the nurse considers to be immoral. This cooperation is called proximate. But other cooperation is quite distant from the evil in question, i.e. the purchase of a shirt whose fabric was woven in a foreign factory whose workers are not being paid a just wage. This cooperation is remote. Reflection on these examples quickly suggests that in reality cooperation takes place on a sliding scale, with some cooperation being very close to the action and some very distant.

Once we have made these distinctions, we can begin to discuss some of the major principles which form the theology of cooperation. Five such principles will be considered here. The first principle is that one may never formally cooperate in evil. Since in formal cooperation a person actually intends the evil, his or her behavior is by definition morally flawed. The second principle is that a person or group may materially cooperate in evil for a sufficient reason. In the case cited above about the person who faces being shot if he or she refuses to drive the gang to their hideout, most people would say that there is a sufficient reason (saving one's life) for driving the gang.

The third principle is that the greater the evil in question, the stronger the motive for material cooperation must be before there can be said to be a sufficient reason. Similarly, the lesser the evil in question, the lesser the motive must be in order to qualify as a sufficient reason. For example it is usually said that if a case can be made for any degree of cooperation related to abortion (e.g. supporting a law which does not fully accord with Catholic teaching), the nature of abortion requires that extremely weighty reasons be present. However, for a case to be made for cooperation in surgical sterilization, the reasons, while still serious, would not have to be as serious as the reasons for abortion-related cooperation. Here I am not trying to suggest which cases for cooperation, if any, can be made for either abortion or sterilization. I am simply suggesting that the nature of these two actions is such that they would call for different levels of strength in the reasons to be proposed as justifications for cooperation.

The fourth principle is that the more closely the material cooperator is involved in the evil, the stronger her or his reason must be in order to justify the cooperation. Likewise, the more remotely the material cooperator is involved in the evil, the lesser his or her reason must be in order to justify the material cooperation. Here we might consider the difference between the role of a nurse who assists a physician in preparing a patient for a surgical procedure which the nurse finds to be morally wrong and the role of a receptionist in the same physician's office who schedules appointments for patients to receive the same procedure. Because the nurse's action is more closely related to the procedure in question, the nurse needs a stronger reason to justify material cooperation. Of course both the nurse and the receptionist have to ask other questions as well. How wrong is the procedure in question? How frequently is this procedure part of the physician's practice? How badly does either the nurse or the receptionist need to keep holding this particular job?[15] As these questions show, the issues raised by the third and fourth principles (seriousness and closeness to the behavior) can interact in a variety of different ways. Once it has been determined that cooperation is material rather than formal, we must be prepared to ask a variety of related questions in order to assess whether material cooperation is justified in a given set of circumstances.

The fifth principle has to do with the amount of scandal which a given instance of material cooperation might cause. If the cooperation is relatively private so that little scandal is likely to be present, or if other factors about a particular cooperation situation make scandal unlikely, relatively lesser reasons will be needed to justify the material cooperation. But if the danger of scandal is high, the reasons for material cooperation will need to be significantly stronger before the cooperation can be justified. Also, in such cases all reasonable measures should be taken to reduce the danger of scandal.

The standard teaching on cooperation has focused very specifically on cooperation in evil. It sometimes happens that persons who disagree with one or another Catholic moral teaching do so in sincere good faith, i.e. because they themselves think that the behavior in question is a morally good action. This fact does not alter the Catholic teaching, nor does it take away the right and responsibility of the church to speak its mind on the issue or issues in question. But in the context of those who sincerely disagree with official church teaching, some authors have suggested that material cooperation is more readily justifiable when the cooperation is given to persons who are in sincere good faith about the behavior in question.[16] This is a very difficult question, and there are signs that the church's magisterium may not want to accept the good faith of others as a basis for material cooperation.[17] On this and related issues, there will need to be continued reflection and awareness of how the tradition of material cooperation develops in the future.

The theology of cooperation has come to the fore in a number of health-related areas in recent years. In many Catholic dioceses in the U.S. there has been a tradition of taking part in United Way campaigns to help raise funding for the church's social programs, even though the United Way also raises funds for some groups which sponsor activities which are not in accord with the teaching of the Catholic Church. In this case it is often argued that the good to be gained from such unified fund drives is significant enough to justify taking part in the unified drives and that the degree of cooperation with the work of the other groups in the fund drive is remote enough not to be a moral issue. This is especially seen to be the case when donors to a unified drive are allowed to specify which charity or charities are to receive their contributions and which charity or charities are prohibited from receiving their contributions. It would also seem that if the Catholic Church is going to cooperate in United Way fund drives, it is necessary that church teaching on the issues in question be clear so that no scandal is given.[18]

Another recent example dealing with material cooperation can be found in reading the Catholic bishops' 1980 statement on the possibility of Catholic hospitals offering material cooperation (through use of their facilities, etc.) in the surgical sterilization of patients. The Catholic bishops were very cautious on this issue, and they stated that cooperation in such sterilizations could not be based on the specific medical facts about the woman seeking the sterilization. Instead, the bishops insisted that the cooperation must be based on factors extrinsic to the facts about the woman. Some have suggested that the bishops were thinking that material cooperation could only be justified on the basis of issues related to the welfare and mission of the hospital. Whatever the exact interpretation, it is important to be aware that the bishops, while very cautious, did not altogether rule out the possibility of material cooperation. In this sense the bishops were faithful to the subtle complexity of the Catholic tradition on material cooperation. The 1975 statement of the Congregation for the Doctrine of the Faith on sterilization was a guide for the bishops as they made their 1980 statement.[19]

This chapter's main point is the excellence of the Catholic tradition on religion and public policy, an excellence which always seeks to make and keep public policy as moral as possible, but an excellence which also recognizes the legitimate autonomy of politics and the need for subtle moral-political judgments on specific issues. Hopefully, this section has shown that the Catholic tradition on material cooperation has a similar subtlety so that the concepts associated with material cooperation may be of significant value when we consider the relationship between religious morality and a complex public policy issue such as health care.

THE CATHOLIC TRADITION ON RELIGION
AND PUBLIC POLICY:
IMPLICATIONS FOR HEALTH CARE REFORM

In view of the tradition we have just reviewed, an obvious question surfaces: What implications can we draw for health care reform from the Catholic approach to religion and public policy? It should go almost without saying that Roman Catholicism's commitment to a moral public policy will call Catholicism to be an articulate proponent of true health care reform. But what about those situations in which official Catholic moral teaching and proposals for health care reform are in conflict or at least appear to be in conflict? I think we can summarize how Catholic moral teaching might approach these conflict situations by dealing with three main types of questions: questions having to do with health care reform proposals which fall short of the goal of universal access to a reasonable level of health care, questions about health care reform proposals which provide services that are opposed to Catholic teaching about sexual morality and abortion, and questions about potential proposals which might disagree with other aspects of Catholic moral teaching. We shall consider each of these three areas of question.

Proposals Which Fall Short of the Goal of Universal Access

In many ways the period in which I have been writing this book has been a period in which there has been a sea change in the attitude of U.S. citizens toward health care reform. While the underlying concern about health care has existed for many years, the early 1990s has suddenly become a time of intense interest in health care reform. The national mood that something must be done grows more and more intense, and the pressure on political leaders to take action becomes ever greater. Because all of this is happening so quickly, there is an excellent chance that some important changes in health care will take place in the first half of the 1990s. But also, because everything is happening so quickly, there is a good chance that the first health care reforms to be made will not be thorough enough, so that there will be a need for a second more rigorously systematic round of health care reform legislation, about five years later, probably during the second half of the 1990s. This same pattern has happened in some other countries in the past,[20] so it would not be surprising for it to happen in the U.S.

All of this can be troubling to Catholic bishops, Catholic theologians, and others (from various religious/moral traditions) who have been thinking about health care reform for years and who have definite moral goals in terms of health care reform. Can such religious/moral leaders support approaches to health care reform which only partly achieve true justice? Can they tolerate health care reforms which do not fully meet the needs of groups such as the poor, racial minorities, women, and children, groups for whom we are called to show a preferential love?

Some examples might be helpful here. One recent proposal suggests that we should reform health care by letting the cost of health insurance be tax deductible. One analysis has shown that this proposal will enable almost a third of those who are currently uninsured (mostly those who work for small businesses which cannot afford health insurance) to be able to buy health insurance. Obviously it would be good that ten million more U.S. citizens have health insurance, but what about the other 25–27 million who are uninsured?[21] If such a tax deduction proposal would make us think we have fixed the problem, and cause us to forget the other uninsured, could those with religious/moral concern for the poor support such a reform?

Another example has to do with the increasing popularity of the "play or pay" approaches to health care reform which we discussed in Chapter 2. Such proposals would surely expand the number of persons who have health insurance, and some "play or pay" plans would come close to universal access. However, because play or pay plans would include a multiplicity of payers for health insurance, it seems that in our culture these plans might very likely involve administrative inefficiencies and higher than necessary health care costs. Thus many would argue that play or pay plans are only a partial answer in the struggle for a truly just national approach to health care delivery.

Other recent proposals call for reduction of support for welfare mothers, especially as they have more and more children.[22] One can certainly understand the concern about teenage pregnancies, etc., and the need to discourage pregnancies on the part of unwed mothers, especially in the cases of those who become pregnant over and over again when they are in need of public assistance. But what about the children who are born through such pregnancies? Would it be just to deny needed assistance to these children, because we do not approve of the behavior of their mothers? Particularly in a religion like Roman Catholicism, with its high commitment to the dignity of the child, could such approaches be seen as real health care reform? Could such approaches be tolerated if they are part of legislation which otherwise contains a great many good aspects?

These kinds of questions are difficult questions, and ultimately each question of this sort will need to be answered on a case by case basis. In general, however, I think the following can be said. If a specific health care reform accomplishes a reasonable but only partial good, and if it is clear that such a proposal is the most that can be accomplished politically at a given time, I think that Catholic bishops and other religious moral leaders could support such a proposal. In their support, such religious leaders would need to make it clear that they are not perfectly satisfied with the legislation, and that, as conditions warrant, they will push for further legislation. All of this goes back to the notion that politics is the art of the possible, and that therefore it can sometimes be reasonable for the Catholic tradition to support legislation which is not yet perfectly moral, if this legislation is the most which is possible at a given time.

To apply this to the examples just cited, I think moral leaders could support tax deductions for the cost of health insurance as a transitional moral step toward true health care reform. Similarly, I could see moral leaders supporting "play or pay" type proposals for health care reform even though they see these proposals as only a transitional moral step toward health care reform. I could not, however, see religious/moral leaders supporting the denial of necessary health care benefits to welfare babies. For me at least, the character of this denial would rule it out, even as a transitional step. In the next chapter, when I discuss my own understanding of a truly just national health care program, I can hopefully make it clearer what it would be reasonable to support as transitional political goals, and what our moral tradition ought to push for as a long term approach to national health care.

Proposals Disagreeing with Catholic Teaching
on Sexual Morality and Abortion

It could well be that some of the proposals for national health care reform in the U.S. will provide a level of access to both counseling and procedures in areas such as contraception, in vitro fertilization, sterilization, and abortion. For those who are committed to the teaching of the Catholic Church, any national health reform which provides access in these areas creates a difficult moral dilemma. On the one hand, national health reform, if it provides health care to the thirty-seven million uninsured persons in the U.S., would be a great good. But on the other hand, the church holds a strong moral stance against contraception, sterilization, and abortion. In dealing with these issues, will Catholic legislators have any choice but to try to use the principles outlined earlier about religion and public policy and about material cooperation? What role will the bishops and other church leaders need to play if such issues come to the fore? I cannot offer complete answers to these questions without knowing exactly which proposals will actually be considered, nor can I provide here a complete account of all the issues related to the church's teaching on sexual morality and abortion. But I do want to make five observations. My first observation will deal with the effect of health care reform proposals on Catholic institutions. The other four will address the relationship of Roman Catholic teaching to the general national dialogue about health care reform.

First, it seems absolutely crucial that no health care reform program require Catholic health care facilities to provide services which are against the teaching of the Catholic Church. For me this would be a violation of the First Amendment, and it could mean the end of Catholic health care in the U.S., at least in areas such as OB-GYN services. Those who would propose such requirements for Catholic hospitals should expect nothing less than all-out opposition from the Catholic bishops and others who are committed to Catholic moral teaching. In the next chapter, when I discuss what I see to be the ideal pattern of health care reform, I will argue on other grounds that health care professionals and institutions ought to be free to choose which services they will provide, how they will maintain quality and price controls, etc. This vision of how health care reform can work best will thus have a

natural coherence with the claim that the religious/moral liberty of
health care institutions ought to be protected.

In saying all this, I am not trying to argue that Catholic health
care institutions will never face situations in which they might legitimately choose to cooperate materially with some practices which run
against Catholic moral teaching. My point rather is that decisions
about material cooperation ought never to be imposed on Catholic
institutions as a matter of government policy. *The Ethical and Religious
Directives for Catholic Health Facilities* are explicitly clear that there are
no circumstances in which a Catholic health facility can provide material cooperation in abortions, and the Catholic Church should have
every right to set such a standard and to follow it without legislative
interference.[23] Some are using the catch-phrase "conscience clause" to
describe the freedom which should be part of any reform laws relating to health care professionals and institutions. Whatever the phrase
to be used, the principle of such freedom is a crucial element in both
our secular and our religious traditions.

Second (and moving from the effect on Catholic institutions to
health care reform in general), the official teaching of the church is
opposed to a number of sexual morality/human life related issues
which might come up in proposals for health care reform. The
church's opposition would touch on issues such as contraception,
sterilization, abortion, and sex education which is not based on premarital abstinence. However, it seems reasonable to argue that each of
these issues does not possess the exact same weight in terms of the
moral evil involved. If this is so, and if it is true that the official church
has limited resources to exercise as a dialogue partner on public policy, it would seem reasonable for the church to focus its opposition on
those health care issues which cause it the greatest level of concern. If
other issues get less emphasis through such an approach, this does not
mean that the church has abandoned its teaching on these other issues. It only means that the church is using its resources to do the best
it can in a given set of historical circumstances.

Third, when we consider the various sexual and reproductive
issues which might be connected with health care reform, it seems fair
to note that on some of these issues the church stands a good chance
of having its views influence the debate about legislation. But on other
issues there would seem to be a rather small possibility that the
church's approach would change the outcome of the debate. For example, there seems to be only a very limited chance that the church's
teaching on contraception will be effective in altering the outcome of
health policy decisions on contraception. Hence it would not seem

that civil law would be the best way for the Catholic Church to promote its teachings on contraception. In this context, Cardinal O'Connor has stated that he does not believe that, except for issues related to abortifacients, any Catholic bishop in the U.S. is in favor of civil legislation against birth control.[24]

However, on an issue such as the preference of abstinence to condom use as an absolutely effective way of preventing someone from becoming HIV positive, the church may be able to get more of a hearing for its viewpoint, even in the area of public policy about sex education.[25] Similarly, on the topic of abortion, we may very well be entering a period in which there will be significant legal restrictions placed on abortion. Even some sociological research which is not committed to the church's viewpoint has indicated that liberal laws on abortion will not continue to be feasible in the U.S. and that laws which place significant restrictions on abortion (even if not completely excluding it) may well be the most likely practical sociological outcome.[26] If it is true that significant legislative change may happen in this area, the church, as a public participant in the dialogue, may be able to exercise a notable influence on that change. Again, if we recall the old notion about politics being the art of the possible, it would seem prudent for the church to spend its energy on political issues where it might be able to effect change, as opposed to issues where it is less likely to have much effect. Such an approach would in no way mean that the teaching church is any less committed to its teachings on those issues which it has chosen not to promote strongly in the political arena.

Fourth, on the specific issue of abortion, Catholic bishops have made it clear that the nature of the abortion issue is such that Catholic legislators should not only oppose abortion morally, but also work to bring about change in existing laws which permit abortion. The bishops' point is that abortion is clearly an issue which involves the public good. Thus the bishops reject any argument which sees abortion as a private issue whose moral status need not concern a Catholic when he or she is acting as a legislator. Both Archbishop John Quinn and Cardinal O'Connor have made a very strong case for the responsibility of the Catholic legislator in working to change abortion legislation.[27] With all this in mind, it seems clear that any Catholic approach to more just health care must proceed from an understanding and acceptance of the Catholic moral and legal teaching on abortion.

Fifth, there remains the question of just how the traditional Catholic concern about the technical feasibility of legislation might interact with specific legislative proposals which provide for universal access to health care while not outlawing all abortions. In his clear statement of the responsibility of the Catholic legislator to work toward the outlawing of abortion, Cardinal O'Connor stated that he recognized that there could be varying political strategies used to seek change in abortion legislation, and he also mentioned three conditions under which a Catholic might support an imperfect bill on abortion. His three conditions were: first, that no better bill be feasible; second, that the bill be better than existing legislation; third, that the bill not preclude further reform in the future. My question is whether these kinds of conditions might ever be met in a health care reform bill which does not outlaw all abortions.[28]

I ask this question in part because, even without making changes in existing abortion law, a health care reform law which provides all people with access to quality health care would already serve to reduce the number of abortions. Sometimes persons seek abortions because of poverty-related reasons, because of fear that they will not be able to provide proper care for a child. If we succeed in health care reform, the negative effect of health care costs on our economy may be significantly ameliorated, perhaps meaning that not so many people will face poverty, unemployment, and other similar factors which make them fear having a child. Even more significantly, with true health care reform, every mother and couple can at least be sure that their child's medical needs will be met, and this will remove one very troubling reason why some persons turn to abortion.

With this context in mind, if a Catholic legislator were convinced that a reform law to guarantee universal health care access would in fact reduce abortions and would only be able to pass if it did not change existing statutes on abortion, could such a legislator reluctantly support such a law, knowing that such a law accomplishes the most good possible at a given time in history? The question might be answered more easily if the legislator felt that laws reducing abortion might be able to pass in the near future, provided that these new laws on abortion were not made part of a health care reform bill. The question might also be easier if the legislator were able to make his or her views on abortion well known in other contexts, and if it were possible for the new health care reform law to contain some explicit provisions aimed at reducing the number of abortions, even if these restrictions did not fully reflect the church's moral teachings.

Complete answers to such questions could only be given in a specific legislative/political situation. In general, however, I believe that it may be possible for circumstances to exist in which these questions could be answered affirmatively, based on the Catholic tradition of technical feasibility, and on Cardinal O'Connor's comments about times when Catholics might support imperfect laws.

In the same sort of context, difficult questions might also arise for Catholic bishops. Might there be political situations related to health care reform in which bishops, at least privately, could choose to respect the good faith of legislators who choose to vote for health care reform legislation which is less than perfect with regard to abortion? Similarly, if health care reform legislation accomplishes much that is good in terms of universal health care access, and if legislative reform on abortion and related issues is simply not politically achievable as part of health care reform, might bishops choose not to publicly oppose such health care reform legislation? In particular, if the bishops' public opposition were to cause health care reform to fail (and still not lead to any changed abortion laws), what course should the bishops take? As with legislators, this question could be a little less difficult if the health care reform legislation included some policies which would reduce the number of abortions even though not doing all the bishops would hope for on this issue. Clearly, only the bishops could answer these questions, and their answer would depend on the specific circumstances. But it is at least possible that these questions could emerge as serious questions.[29]

Other Possible Conflicts

The two issues we have so far cited—proposals which do not go far enough to reform health care and proposals which are not in full accord with Catholic teaching on sexual morality and abortion—probably capture the bulk of the issues around which Catholic moral teaching and health care reform initiatives might conflict. But there are other possible conflictual areas as well. Even though the euthanasia initiative in the state of Washington was defeated in November 1991, such initiatives are likely to appear again in other places, and there might be a potential for some mixing of health care reform proposals and euthanasia initiatives. Also, because the interest in genetic research is so high, some health care reform proposals might include funding for genetic research whose methods and/or objectives would be opposed to Catholic moral values.

On these matters, and any other similar issues which come to the fore, I have two main thoughts. First, because these issues would be fairly new factors in the debate about health care reform, I think they could be opposed strongly with little political impact on health care reform itself. Indeed, I would hope that the debate about euthanasia would not become admixed with the debate about health care reform, and I think that Catholics and others concerned about euthanasia should not only express their opposition but also urge that this issue not become linked up with health care reform. Second, I think that the fundamental soundness of the Catholic tradition on religious morality and public policy is such that the principles of this tradition can be successfully applied in practice to any new moral issues which might enter into the debate about health care reform. None of us can foresee all of the twists and turns which the process of health care reform may take over the next few years. But with a strategy of maintaining clear moral values and sensitively applying them in the concrete political world, I think religious and moral thinking can make momentous contributions to the national effort for true health care reform.

Chapter 8

WHAT SHOULD A REFORMED HEALTH CARE SYSTEM LOOK LIKE?

In this book we have looked at the crisis in the U.S. health care, at the major political options to address the crisis, at theological and moral resources to help us face the crisis, and at the role of church teaching in debates about public policy. All of these matters have led up to this book's final question: What should a reformed health care system look like? As a theologian I must acknowledge that there are some details in terms of health care economics and medical standards which I am not competent to address. Nonetheless, I think the topics considered in this book provide a basis for a sound overall description of a revised health care system for the U.S. I will present my description of a new U.S. health care system by offering fifteen conclusions. Some of the conclusions will recapitulate issues taken up in earlier chapters. I thought it best to pull all the issues together at this point so as to give an integrated outline of the main features of a new health care system for the U.S.[1]

FIRST CONCLUSION:
THE DEMAND OF JUSTICE

Universal access to a reasonable level of health care in the U.S. is necessary as a matter of justice and human rights.

In recent times, political pressures have mounted to the point that some kind of change in our health care seems to be inevitable. What needs to be remembered is that the need for health care reform rests on much deeper foundations than practical political necessity. Once we accept the fundamental theory of distributive justice, it follows that every citizen ought to have access to decent health care. The fact that nearly one quarter of our citizens are either uninsured or underinsured stands as a moral outrage, especially when we compare the U.S. with other western countries. Arrogant claims that we have the best health care in the world and attacks on the health care systems of other countries seem to stem from a failure of imagination and from a moral blindness.

It is crucial that we recognize the justice/rights foundation of the call to health care reform so that we take the issue seriously enough and adopt truly adequate solutions. Because of the growing political pressure for change, there is a danger that partial, politically attractive health care reforms will be enacted which will not be truly adequate and which will only be the occasion for more complaints and more changes later on. To a degree this is inevitable, and the move toward a fully just U.S. health care system will probably occur in several phases over a period of years. But the more we can keep our attention centered on the justice issues which are at the core of health care reform, the more effectively we can move to true reform, even if it all does take time. Only when universal access to a decent level of health care has been accomplished will the U.S have achieved a genuinely just health care system.

Just health care is necessary so that we can have a good, hopeful, and stable society. If many persons feel that their health care needs will not be met, these persons will lose hope in terms of future plans for education, family building, productive employment, etc. This loss of hope will lead to a society which is less confident in its ability to move into the future, a society in which people are more hostile to one another. Even today one reads that many people in the U.S. think that our country's best days are past and that we are in a state of decline. I cannot judge how true these pessimistic assessments are, but it does seem certain that the lack of access to health care is a major factor in the pessimism of our times. If we want U.S. society to be a stable and flourishing society, it must be a just society. No doubt there are many issues which contribute to the building of a just society. In our particular historical era, universal access to health care stands as a crucial building block for a just society.

SECOND CONCLUSION:
HEALTH CARE REFORM A PRAGMATIC NECESSITY

Universal health care access can be delivered in a fashion which is more efficient and cost effective than our présent piecemeal system. A more efficient system of health care delivery will benefit both persons who need health care and the U.S. economy as a whole.

No health care delivery system is or will be perfect. I believe, however, that there is clear evidence that the present U.S. system is grossly inefficient in terms of its basic financing structure, in terms of its complex network of private insurance carriers, and in terms of its multifaceted delivery system which is confusing to so many people. Even if our two economies and cultures are not exactly the same, I think the statistics about the administrative cost for health care in Canada offer a compelling argument that a more efficient and cost effective system of delivery is possible.[2] Even the relatively effective administrative performance of the U.S. Medicare system, with all its problems, shows that there can be a more efficient approach to health care financing than an approach based on the work of 1,500 private health insurance companies.

There is a great deal of concern today about the overall state of the U.S. economy and about the difficulty that the U.S. faces in marketing products which have a price and quality that are comparable to the price and quality of similar products produced in other countries. Surely there are many factors which help explain the difficulties of the U.S. economy, factors such as our country's high cost for defense, our desire for high wages, and the inadequate education of some workers. There is little doubt, however, that the high cost of health care is a significant factor pressuring our economy in a negative direction. If we can come up with a good program of health care reform, such a program may have benefits which go far beyond health care itself.

The first conclusion argued for health care reform as a matter of justice; it called for health care reform so that we can be the sort of people we want to be. The second conclusion calls for the same reform as a pragmatic matter, as an issue which can bring about more efficient health care along with potential benefits to the U.S economy and to the prestige to the U.S. in the world at large. As a theologian, I think the first conclusion is more important than the second, but, as often happens, approaches to a just society offer real, pragmatic benefits. The old saying is that good morality and good medicine go together. Today I think we can expand that saying and assert that good morality, good medicine, just access to health care, and a strong national economy can all go together.

THIRD CONCLUSION: PREFERENCE FOR A SINGLE PAYER SYSTEM

Of all the proposed initiatives for health care reform, those initiatives which call for a national single payer insurance system seem to be the most just and to offer that highest potential for genuine long term health care reform.

This is probably the most controversial of my conclusions, so I will need to take a little more time to defend it. There are two main reasons why I think the single payer system has the highest potential for true health care reform. First of all, at this time in U.S. history, the single payer approach has the best chance to fulfill the traditional norms of distributive justice. Earlier, when talking about distributive justice, I argued that maximum distributive justice would be achieved when a strong basic standard of care was agreed on for every different medical situation, and when everyone in a specific medical situation has access to that same basic standard. To me it seems inevitable that if we continue a mix of private and public insurance systems, different standards of care will develop in different health care settings, and that certain groups—most likely the poor and racial minorities—will continue to have access to a lower basic standard of care than will the rest of society. If this happens, our health care system will continue to be unstable and in need of further reform.

Secondly, I think the single payer approach can be more efficient and cost effective than any other approach to health care delivery. If we continue with a multiplicity of health care insurance systems, it seems certain that there will be duplication of services, ongoing public confusion about what health care services are really needed, more complex health care administration structures, and, most importantly, higher health care costs. Even a program such as that proposed by Senator Kerrey, which comes close to a single payer system, still contemplates a multiplicity of insurors and therefore invites a continuation of the problems which already beset the U.S. health care system.[3]

In terms of the fears related to a single payer system, many people in our society have a natural—and sometimes well placed—fear of entrusting government with too much stewardship of human services. No doubt a certain Lutheran pessimism about government has its place. However, when we consider other segments of the Christian tradition, both Protestant and Catholic, both Augustinian and Thomistic, there seems to be more reason to trust in government to help us solve difficult social problems. Throughout this book we have talked about the Thomistic natural law tradition with its confidence—admittedly a sober confidence—in the role of government. For me at least, it is hard not to think that the Thomistic tradition and the principles of modern Catholic social teaching are such as to argue for a substantial level of government involvement in an issue as complex as modern health care delivery.

In Protestant America, the greatest of all the moral thinkers was Reinhold Niebuhr. In the early 1930s he wrote his famous book *Moral Man and Immoral Society*.[4] In the book Niebuhr argued that collective entities by their nature contain more evil than individual persons. Niebuhr's insight, which is surely true, gives all of us a natural hesitancy about placing too much power over individual lives in the hands of governments, especially large governments. But Niebuhr did not argue in *Moral Man* (or in his later works) against a substantial role for government in addressing social problems. Instead, and in the spirit of Augustine, he was concerned that we recognize government for what it is and develop political strategies appropriate to counteract the negative tendencies of government.[5] Later on in life he even argued that the difference between individuals (who are also sinners needing to be kept under control) and collectives is not as great as he had suggested in *Moral Man*. He even suggested that if he were writing *Moral Man* again he would title it "The not so moral man and his even less moral communities."[6] To me it seems that we have seen a lot of not so moral things going on in the delivery of modern health care. A strong governmental reform such as the single payer system may be the most effective way out of the morass.

Besides the fear of too large a role for government, the other main fear connected with the single payer system is that it will involve the collection of more tax monies. While this is true, it should be remembered that much of the additional tax money to be collected will be a replacement of the money which many large employers pay for private insurance plans. Some of the money will come from taxes on smaller businesses which would like to be able to provide health insurance for their employees but which cannot now do so because private insurance is too expensive. In addition, there is the crucial fact that, if properly managed, a single payer system will have the potential to save us all a great deal of money in health care expenditures, especially as the years go by. Recall, for instance, the projection of Evans and Lomas that at the present time the U.S. could save $100 billion a year through a single payer system.[7] Congressman Russo, relying on the Government Accounting Office, recently projected that this year's administrative savings could be $67 billion.[8] If the use of taxation can actually save money in the long run while providing universal access to health care, I fail to see a substantive argument against this kind of tax policy. In the end it may well happen that a sound approach to health care reform, particularly if it is coupled with other strategies for productive growth, will enhance the tax base of the entire U.S. economy, so that over the years the tax burden of just health care will be manageable in a reasonable fashion.

I want to emphasize that, in taking my stand for the single payer system, I am speaking about the United States at this time in history. Without doubt there are other countries, especially in western Europe, that have had substantial success with "play or pay" approaches to health care delivery. These countries are working from a considerably different philosophy of both business and insurance than what now exists in the U.S., so that it would be unthinkable for persons to be excluded from health insurance because of high risk, etc. Insurance companies in these countries operate with strong governmental controls and with a high sense of covenantal responsibility toward the people they insure.[9] If the U.S. philosophy of insurance evolves over a period of time, other approaches to health care delivery may well deserve to be tried. But as of now, the single payer approach seems clearly to be the best moral option available to the U.S. for the delivery of health care. I realize that the single payer approach may eliminate the current jobs of some persons in insurance and related fields. Some of these persons will move to relocated employment as part of a national insurance system. All reasonable efforts must be made to help persons affected by a new health system to find suitable work, but the priority of the common good argues that the first task is to find a just health care system for the U.S. as a whole.

In reflecting on the single payer system, it has been hard not to think about health care delivery as having some parallels to national defense since both are such enormous factors in our national economy and have so much impact on the quality of life in the U.S. For this reason it is interesting to reflect on the financial history and administration of our national defense system throughout the years. Until after World War II, defense was administered by separate armed services, with both Army and Navy having cabinet-rank secretaries, with sometimes inadequate communications and planning, and with some needless overlapping of equipment, capabilities, etc. When President Truman first proposed integrating the armed services, the idea was anathema to many, as it was thought that we simply could not afford to lose the separate traditions of the armed services. Several years were necessary before Mr. Truman's plans could come to fruition.[10] Today, however, most Americans would find it inconceivable for the U.S. not to have a unified defense department. With important differences which we will see as we move along, I think the case for a unified national financial management of health care is as compelling as the case for a unified national defense system. To use the traditional Catholic language, the financial administration of health care seems clearly to be a situation in which the demands of justice are such that both the principle of subsidiarity and the principle of socialization require a greater governmental role.

Some might argue that since defense exists to protect our national security, i.e. to protect the U.S. from potential destruction by its enemies, no other issue can be compared to defense. Hence, no other issue can justify such a large scale of direct financial management. I think it can be argued that lack of adequate access to health care is an issue which threatens very much to destabilize the U.S. Also, our economic viability as a nation is threatened because of the uncontrolled and ever spiraling cost of health care. From this perspective, health care can clearly be said to be a national security issue which calls for national financial management.

For a single payer system to work, some kind of a national commission on health care will need to be established. Much work will need to be done on the description and functions of such a commission, but some of its key duties will be to establish a package of basic health benefits to be covered for all citizens, to advise congress on the amount of money which needs to be spent, to set priorities for health care expenditure, to establish national quality and cost management standards, and to set appropriate allocation formulas for each state. Such a commission would need to have members with a range of expertise, and it is critical that it be set up so as to be truly sensitive to the health care needs of all the American people. Because of the pivotal role of such a commission, it is hard not to think about the time-honored method of presidential appointment and senatorial approval as the means of placing members on the commission.

To close this section on the moral priority of a single payer system, I want to add two disclaimers. First, a national single payer system need not exclude some citizens seeking some non-covered health services to be paid for on some other basis. Such services need not be excluded provided that they do not prevent the single payer system from offering a high enough level of coverage to assure most people in the U.S. that their essential health care needs are met. We will see more on this point in the seventh conclusion. The second disclaimer is that, in terms of practical politics, the priority of the single payer system does not mean that the use of other transitional approaches to reform should be excluded. It may be politically more feasible so get some other reform option (such as play or pay?) in place before the national consensus is ready to turn to a single payer system. If this happens, such another option may both accomplish some intermediate health care good and be a useful learning experience which will help the single payer system be even better once its time comes. For me at least, the long term trend towards a single payer option seems inevitable, at least in the current cultural context of the United States.

FOURTH CONCLUSION:
A ROLE FOR THE STATES

In the United States, a single payer national health insurance system ought to be administered by the states.

There are differences in the health care needs of our different states because of factors such as climate, industries which are present, and predominant ethnic or racial groups which tend to have certain health problems. Also, there can be differences in the cost of living from state to state, meaning that just wages for health care workers, especially lower paid workers, can vary from state to state. Even within a given state, there can be differences on all these matters from region to region. Therefore, even though the basic financing structure and standard setting for health care should occur at the federal level, the individual states, relying on the principle of subsidiarity, ought to have the freedom to apply the national standards to their own needs. This would mean that the federal government would allocate the tax funds for health care to the states who would then have the responsibility of reimbursing the health care providers. This role for the states can serve as an important check against the federal government's having too much control over the delivery of health care services. The individual state might choose to handle the disbursement of the health care funds by establishing a state agency, or the individual state might choose to contract with a private entity to handle the disbursement process. But the states would not be free to contract with a variety of local entities which would be free to offer competing reimbursement plans. The experience of countries which have used a single payer system shows that such a system can be substantially more efficient than multiple payer systems while maintaining a standard of good quality medical care. In my judgment, this is a fact which cannot be ignored.

FIFTH CONCLUSION:
THE NEED FOR PRIVATE DELIVERY OF CARE

Even though the reimbursement for health care services and the setting of health care standards need to take place nationally, the delivery of health care (by physicians, hospitals, and related services) should remain largely in private hands.

Like the third conclusion, this is a pivotally important notion for the future of quality health care in the United States. For the individual patient to be sure that he or she is getting truly quality care, the patient should remain free, within reasonable limits, to choose his or her own sources of health care delivery. For the individual doctor, hospital, HMO, etc., to continue to be motivated to offer the best possible care, the doctor, hospital, HMO, etc., should have to compete for patients, even though they know that they are assured payment for those patients they do succeed in attracting. To say this in another way, the free market ought to continue to exist in terms of the delivery of health care services.[11] I am not claiming here that a private delivery system will always be successful in delivering quality care to individual patients. But the value of private delivery is significant enough that the compelling arguments for the unification of the financing of health care do not apply to the delivery of health care services. The Catholic Health Association of the United States describes all this as "Unitary Payment" and "Pluralistic Delivery."[12]

Once it is stipulated that there should be a pluralism of providers competing for patients, I think it becomes clear that I am not proposing socialized medicine as such. In the British system, the government owns many hospitals and is very strongly in the business of delivering health care as well as financing it. This is what I understand as socialized medicine. In a reformed U.S. system, while the government would finance universal access to health care, the health care system itself would primarily be composed of private hospitals and doctors. This would not rule out government ownership of some hospitals (which already happens), but government ownership of services would not be the primary means of health care delivery. All this would mean that a new health care system for the U.S. would be much more like the Canadian system than like the British system. All of this would also mean that my earlier parallel of health care and national defense would apply to the financing of health care but not to the delivery of health care.

In Chapter 7 I argued that the retention of a private system for the delivery of health care would be good for Catholic health care institutions because it would assure that these institutions could continue to operate under the *Ethical and Religious Directives* which have been promulgated by the bishops for Catholic health care facilities in the U.S. Here I am arguing that the retention of privately owned hospitals and other health services would help accomplish the even larger human good of assuring maximum quality care and maximum respect for the dignity and worth of each individual patient. Sadly, there are as many unique ways to be sick as there are people who get sick. A system in which actual delivery decisions remain in private hands is more likely to assure that the true human and health care needs of each person are met in the best way possible.

To say that the delivery of health care services would remain largely in private hands does not mean that the private purveyors of health care would be totally free of government controls. Obviously through the national and state health boards there would be policies to regulate costs and charges, priorities in terms of what most needs to be provided, and so forth. In point of fact, private hospitals and doctors are already dealing with a great deal of government regulation through the Medicare system and a number of other mechanisms. Some of the current regulations can be confusing and overlapping, a situation which can hopefully be rectified through a unified national health insurance system.

SIXTH CONCLUSION:
THE INTEGRATION OF PRIVATE SERVICES

The private providers of health care need to make all reasonable efforts to integrate their services into wholistic networks so that the individual health care consumer can avoid dealing with a variety of disjointed health care services.

At the bedside I sometimes deal with a dying patient who is being cared for by a number of doctors who do not seem to be in good communication with one another about the patient. All the more so, there are great numbers of people who deal with many disparate health care providers. Such patients can often be unsure about what they really need, about where to turn next for health care. Particularly when a patient needs to make a transition from one health care setting to another (e.g. from a hospital to a nursing home or vice versa), the patient and his or her family may be very uncertain as to how to work all this out. In a fragmented system such as ours, some important and cost effective health care services (such as preventive care) are too often left out altogether.

To remedy these problems, it would be very helpful if the disparate private providers of health care services would unite themselves into networks. Then a patient could turn to such a network and have confidence that all of her or his health care needs will be addressed in a coherent fashion. In this context the experience of the effective HMO health care settings is very instructive. In a good HMO, the satisfaction of the patients occurs precisely because the wholistic needs of the patient are addressed in an integrated context.

In its setting of parameters for health care reform, the Catholic Health Association places great stress on this notion of integrated delivery networks.[13] The CHA even suggests that a health care provider not be qualified to receive payment from the national health insurance system unless the provider is part of an integrated delivery network. To ensure true competition the CHA would want there to be at least two integrated delivery networks accessible to consumers in every part of every state. In connection with its emphasis on networking, the CHA also makes some very helpful suggestions about unified national standards for medical record keeping.

I understand the concerns behind the CHA approach to integrated networks, and I certainly think that the policies of the national and state health boards should be designed to provide positive incentives for the development of integrated delivery networks. However, I would not favor membership in an integrated delivery network as a necessary qualification for a health care provider to be eligible to receive national health insurance funds as payment for services rendered. It seems to me that at times a small independent provider may come up with a really good idea for health care delivery—an idea which meets some people's needs—which the delivery networks in an area are not willing to accept. One thinks about the many health care settings which have emerged in the recent past such as hospices for dying AIDS patients and storefront clinics in poor neighborhoods. These settings would surely be part of delivery networks, but if imaginative new health care settings should emerge, I would like to give settings a chance to flourish, even if integrated delivery networks are not yet ready to include them.

SEVENTH CONCLUSION:
ADEQUATE COVERAGE FOR ALL

In addition to focusing on integration, the level of coverage provided by a national health insurance system should be able to meet the genuine health care needs of most people most of the time.

In terms of the exact details of what should be covered by a national health insurance system, there are many issues which are not strictly within the province of a theologian to address. The question about the level of coverage is partly a matter of economics, of how much we as a nation can afford to spend on health care, especially in light of our other national needs such as defense, education, transportation, housing, and human development. The question about coverage is also partly medical: Which kinds of treatments are most truly indicated medically in given sets of health circumstances? These economic and medical questions will be in a continuing process of change, so that the coverage level of a national health insurance system will be in a process of constant reassessment.

What can be said theologically and morally is that the coverage level needs to be adequate to meet the needs of most people most of the time. Otherwise the national insurance system will be constantly unstable. People would try to avoid using it. The effort to seek other sources of health care by those who could afford to do so would become so prevalent that our economy would continue to be under the same health care related stress which it faces today. It is certainly clear that no national insurance system will satisfy everyone all of the time. But if poll takers such as Louis Harris are correct, national systems such as Canada's have achieved a high enough level of satisfaction to work effectively.[14]

In terms of the areas which a national system should cover, the following general areas ought to be included: primary care physicians, preventive care programs, prenatal and postnatal care for mothers and children, hospitalization, specialists, prescriptions, dental services, substance abuse services, mental health services, and long term care (including services such as nursing homes and home care programs). All human persons have a fundamental dignity on the basis of their common humanity and status as children of God. The general areas which I have just listed strike me as the fundamental or basic health care services which all persons ought to receive because of their shared human dignity. These services are the areas in which all persons have a right of access to a fundamental package of similar treatments, regardless of any other factors.

As to exactly what should be covered in these areas, I refer to my earlier point about the need for health economists and medical experts to work out the best specifics possible. I placed primary care physicians first on the list because in many situations they will be the channel through which patients access the other levels of covered services. Also, even within a national insurance system, I would not completely rule out measures such as a small copayment for office visits and prescriptions if it could be shown that such measures helped control costs, and provided that such measures were designed so as not to exclude the poor.

EIGHTH CONCLUSION:
CARE FOR THE POOR AND MULTICULTURAL GROUPS

While the standard of care for the poor and related groups such as racial, linguistic, and cultural minorities should be the same as for everyone else, special procedural measures should be adopted to ensure that the poor and related groups are able to make appropriate use of the universal access available to them through a national health insurance system.

In Chapter 6 I argued that the standard of justice in terms of health care services should be the same for all people. At this level of basic standard, I do not see a place for a preferential option for the poor. However, in terms of applying the standard in practice, it seems certain that factors such as fear, lack of education, a sense of isolation, etc., may tend to keep the poor from seeking the health care which would be theirs by law in a national single payer system. Thus a national health insurance system must include special programs of outreach to inform the poor of their rights and draw them to seek the health care which they need. It is at this level, which I call the procedural level, that I believe a case can be made for a preferential option for the poor. Such a procedural preferential option is right not only from the viewpoint of justice but also from the viewpoint of economic efficiency. If we can get the poor and other alienated groups to seek health care earlier, their care will be less expensive, and they will be in a better position to be productive members of society.

I mention other groups besides the poor because of my conviction that the fear of seeking needed health care can come from a variety of sources other than sheer poverty. In my role as a medical ethicist, some of my most heart-rending experiences in individual cases have involved persons from very different cultural settings and language backgrounds, which made it very difficult for them to address what appropriate health care might be in a complex set of circumstances. These experiences have convinced me that any special outreach to deliver health care must be multicultural as well as focused on the poor.

NINTH CONCLUSION:
ACCEPTANCE OF DEATH AS PART OF LIFE

For a national health care system to be truly effective, we need to build a new national consensus on the meaning of death and life, a consensus which will help us to avoid overtreatment without sliding toward active euthanasia. For the building of such a consensus, the moral tradition of Roman Catholicism is an especially rich resource. The achievement of this consensus will help us to practice true stewardship in the delivery of health care.

We reviewed these matters in detail in Chapters 3 and 4, so here the point is more simple. If the United States is going to be able to afford to provide universal access to health care, we are going to need to find ways to prevent vast amounts of money and health care resources from being invested in technological interventions which are not truly proportionate to the needs of individual patients. To avoid these overtreatment problems, we need a revitalized understanding of who we are as human persons and what it means for us to be a moral community committed to the common good. We need to be able to honestly face up to death when it is truly time to die. Facing death is ultimately a religious/moral problem which is why the resources of religious traditions such as Roman Catholicism can be so valuable as we struggle to address the meaning of death in human life.

The economic impact of decisions not to overtreat is obvious in the context of our national health care needs. But the economic question should never obscure the even deeper question of what is truly good for the human person. My conviction is that overtreatment is contrary to the dignity of the human person. It is for this reason—human dignity—that we should make decisions not to overtreat. But once we have acted on such a human dignity basis, we can rejoice that in the providence of God we now have more health care resources to use in cases where the use of the resources will be truly proportionate.

The stress on the problem of overtreatment should not obscure the fact that there are undertreatment problems as well. Indeed, in many respects this entire book has been written because of concern about the millions who are not getting enough medical treatment. The concern about overtreatment should also not lead us toward euthanasia. But with all these cautions, overtreatment is an issue which must be overcome as we journey toward just health care for the U.S.

TENTH CONCLUSION:
EMPHASIS ON PREVENTIVE CARE

For a national renewal of health care delivery to be truly efficient, there must be a strong focus on preventive health care both by individuals and by families, and through appropriate public efforts.

Because of the amazing scientific accomplishments of modern medicine, too many people in the U.S. have been lulled into thinking that medicine can fix every health problem once it arises. In the ninth conclusion we spoke about the need for a new attitude toward death and life. A similar new attitude or spirit of conversion is called for in terms of concentrating on preventive care. Individuals and families need to work at preventive care through the development of good health habits. Public health programs also need to emphasize preventive care through steps such as health education, immunization, and environmental protection. This new focus on preventive care is necessary not only for the good of individuals, but also for the common good so that the community's health care resources will not be used unnecessarily. In looking at U.S. culture today, one sometimes gets the impression that many persons have lost the sense of self discipline which marked so many traditional societies. The result is an emphasis on instant gratification instead of on long-term goals. From this perspective, a focus on preventive health care may have benefits for the U.S. which go beyond the simple fact of conserving health care resources. Steady daily practices to enhance one's health have the potential to be an important kind of renewal of the human spirit, both for individuals and for the community as a whole.

ELEVENTH CONCLUSION:
FACING UP TO RATIONING

In addition to achieving all possible management efficiencies through the avoidance of overtreatment and through preventive care, a truly effective national health insurance system must face up to the fact that it will have to set limits on how much beneficial health care it is possible for a sound society to offer its citizens.

Like conclusions three and five, this is a critically important issue. We live in a finite world in which it is not possible to achieve all goods at the same time. The need for limits in health care becomes all the more clear when we consider that health care is only one of the vital goods which society must be sure that its citizens can attain. The human need for health care must be interrelated with other crucial human goods such as education, housing, and national security. Like the question of beneficial treatment vis-à-vis unbeneficial overtreatment, this theme of health care resources as finite raises ultimate questions about who we are as human persons and about what is truly possible for us as we seek to live together on this planet. The finitude question is thus a religious/moral question upon which theological insights from the various religious traditions should be brought to bear.

In my judgment the greatest weakness of the earlier single payer health care systems (such as Canada's) is that they have not really addressed the theme of human finitude with its implication that some rationing decisions will have to be made in the health care area. I think that Canada's great success has stemmed from the fact that it found a health care setting which has proven to be so much more efficient than the U.S.'s haphazard system. But even in Canada it is becoming more clear that its highly cost effective approach is going to have to confront the issue of rationing. If an effective single payer system can be linked with sound policies which establish genuinely human boundaries to health care efforts, then there is a real chance that true health care reform can succeed. The Oregon plan for Medicaid funding may have some flaws, but if the basic instinct behind Oregon can be combined with the insights gained from a country like Canada, I think health care reform will at last be on the right road.

In Chapter 6 I described the main moral criteria which a health care rationing plan must meet if it is to be just. I will not repeat these criteria here, but I do want to stress the enormous importance of enabling all people to participate as much as possible in decisions about health care rationing. Because we are talking about facing up to the realities of death, life, and human finitude, we are really talking about the need for a true conversion of human hearts and human minds, about the kind of conversion that comes about through prayer and sober reflection.[15] If rationing is simply imposed on people without the creation of a context for true conversion, rationing will not work. My hope would be that churches, synagogues, schools, health care centers, community service organizations, and other similar groups will all become places for true dialogue about the nature of health care and about the need for limits in light of the true character of the human condition.

TWELFTH CONCLUSION: ACCEPTABLE AND UNACCEPTABLE BASES FOR RATIONING

In facing the question of rationing potentially beneficial medical care, society needs to focus on the burdens involved in offering certain types of medical service and on the medical circumstances of the patients to whom such services may or may not be offered. Other factors about patients should not be a basis for any rationing decision.

Clearly the basic rationing question has to do with the pressure which the effort to provide some elaborate modern medical services can place upon the common good. Thus it is appropriate to ask questions such as how difficult it is to provide certain services, both in terms of cost and in terms of medical expertise which might be channeled in other directions. It is also appropriate to ask what losses of other notable human goods will result from the effort to provide these medical services. In the same vein, it is proper to ask about the true necessity and moral goodness of particular medical services. We can also ask about whether the way in which we go about providing some services compromises our character as a people. Some might argue, for instance, that we have been unable to develop a prejudice-free process for allocating scarce organs for transplantation, and that it might be morally better not to transplant scarce organs until we can find a truly moral process for allocating them.

All these questions relate to the burdens—economic, personnel, moral, etc.—which society can face as it tries to provide beneficial medical services. Another crucial line of questioning relates to the degree of benefit which a given person might gain from receiving a burdensome type of medical service. To my way of thinking this is a much trickier question, because as human persons we are unique, and because a failure to recognize the uniqueness of each one of us can be a denial of human dignity. I do think that there are some circumstances in which the benefit of a burdensome technology for a given person can be shown to be very limited on *medical* grounds. This clear medical limit might be part of the basis (along with society's true need to use its resources elsewhere) for a decision not to provide such a medical treatment. I think it is much more problematic, however, to argue that beneficial treatment might be denied because of other human considerations about the patient in question.

In this context, the question of older age is a particularly vexing issue. There are ways in which aging is a medical reality which gives focus to how burdensome and how effective a technological intervention may or may not be for a given person. But it is also true that age is more than a medical fact. People's later years can be a precious and very worthwhile part of life, and older people can often be notable contributors to the common good and to the lives of their families and friends. We need to reflect on the fact that physical health can be very different from one seventy year old person to the next, or from one eighty year old person to the next. There is also the fact that women as a group live longer than men, making it seem unjust to try to apply one age-related rationing standard to both sexes.

For all these reasons I am opposed to the use of age alone as a criteria for health care rationing decisions. When age can be linked with a series of other specific medical facts about a given person in his or her seventies, eighties or beyond, then I believe this series of factors, including age, could be a just basis for a rationing decision. Gerontological studies need to help us learn more and more about aging as a medical fact to help us make good decisions in this area.

In my discussions with peers in ethics, I find a very high regard for the work of Daniel Callahan in terms of his asking the right questions and getting us pointed in very helpful directions in terms of health care rationing. There is, however, a strong sentiment that Callahan may have focused too simply on age as a criterion for health care rationing, especially in the book *Setting Limits*. Herein I am not trying to abandon Callahan's concern about age, but I am trying to link it with other factors, so that age alone would not automatically exclude the use of some technologies. I do agree that the older a person gets, the more likely it is that the person's overall medical condition may exclude some interventions. My point is to always keep overall medical condition in the picture along with age.[16]

Another very difficult moral question related to rationing is the question of setting priorities vis-à-vis persons with very rare burdensome diseases. If we agree that human finitude makes it impossible to develop new approaches or cures for all diseases at the same time, it seems reasonable to argue that the rarity of a disease may make medical research less of a priority than it would be for other diseases. However, if we take a stance of generally excluding rare diseases from medical research, we run a real risk of dehumanizing persons with rare diseases, of denying the true dignity and equality of such fellow human beings. There are no simple answers to the dilemma posed by rare diseases, and even when we cannot cure such diseases we must always care for persons who have them. I would argue that at least some of our annual efforts at medical research and development ought to be devoted to rare diseases. Along with the provision of good care, such a step will help make it clear that, even if we should and do omit some possible work on rare diseases, we will not be writing rare diseases and people who suffer with them out of the health care equation.

THIRTEENTH CONCLUSION:
THE GLOBALIZATION OF HEALTH CARE DELIVERY

While the focus of this book has been on U.S. health care, the world as a whole must quickly begin to address the question of the just delivery of health care everywhere on earth.

Two key factors lead me to assert this conclusion. First, if we study issues related to life and health on a global basis, we find quickly and sadly that there are still places where people's life expectancy remains in the high forties, i.e. places where the standard of health care is in many respects a century behind the standard of care available in the developed countries.[17] This raises profound questions about distributive health care justice for people in certain countries. It also raises questions about our ability to have a world of true peace. The danger is that those who lack basic justice in health care and in areas of basic human need will find it attractive to resort to war as a means of achieving the justice they want. Especially at a time when the possession of nuclear weapons may spread to some of the small and disadvantaged countries, there can be a very great danger from wars that may be started by those who lack access to basic justice in areas such as health care. So even though the health care access problem is critical within the U.S., for the sake of peace and justice we quickly need to move to a global perspective on this issue.

The other factor which raises growing concern about the global delivery of health care has to do with the concept of sovereignity. The whole notion of sovereign independent nation states seems to be moving into a period of significant change as part of the process which is generating the emergence of the so called "new world order."[18] The idea of sovereignity has its roots in the person of the sovereign, the king. In recent centuries the concept of sovereignity has attached itself to the modern nation state which we have become accustomed to calling a sovereign state (with a right to declare war, establish national laws, issue currency, etc.). But much in this current notion of sovereignty may be changing. Consider, for instance, the situation of the European Economic Community in which many of the functions traditionally ascribed to the sovereign state are being absorbed by the European Economic Community. Consider also the situation of all the republics which have recently emerged out of the former Soviet Union. These republics may not end up possessing all the attributes which we have traditionally connected with sovereignty. In light of these trends (and even of the Persian Gulf war), the role of world government through the U.N. and related organizations may become more and more prominent as we move into the twenty-first century. I admit that it is too early to predict all the outcomes of the current international political-economic scene. But it may well be that in a fairly short number of years it will be simply unthinkable politically to consider an issue like just health care delivery on anything other than a global basis. I think this makes it all the more imperative that the U.S. get its own health care act together so that it can play a significant role in any future reorganization of the worldwide delivery of health care.

FOURTEENTH CONCLUSION:
INTERNATIONAL PLANNING FOR RESEARCH

The cost of research and development to generate new health care technologies needs to be shared by the world as a whole, and especially by all those countries whose economies are such that they can contribute to the cost of health care research.

In this book we have noted the truly wonderful things which modern medicine can do, but we have not looked extensively at the issue of health care research which is a very costly undertaking. In terms of our earlier discussion of health care rationing, it should be clear that we need to establish priorities for health care research and that maybe some health research projects will not be possible at a given time in history. But a sound approach to health care delivery must continue a significant level of medical research, and the cost of this research will necessarily be high.

In this context, and even granting that there are some genuine ethical questions to be asked about the pricing policies of groups such as drug companies, I think it is not unfair to state that one major reason why medicine in the U.S. has been so costly is that the prices charged for the use of certain medical services are designed so as to recover the costs of the research which was needed to develop these services. This is the case for drug costs, and for the cost of the use of sophisticated devices such as MRIs. I also think it is fair to say that at least part of the reason why some countries have been able to keep their health costs down is that these countries have been able to take advantage of research breakthroughs without paying for research to the extent that other countries, especially the U.S., pay for research. Early in the book I mentioned that one reason why U.S. automobile prices are so high is that U.S. automakers pay such a large amount for health care. At least part of the health care cost for a U.S. auto is health care research cost.

I am not sure about the best mechanism to deal with this issue, and there are obvious links to the issues of sovereignty and international economic cooperation which I mentioned in the thirteenth conclusion. But it may well be that some sort of large international health research fund administered by the U.N. and paid for by all financially able countries, in accord with their different financial abilities, will be necessary to help keep any one country from bearing a disproportionate cost for health care research. As with physicians and hospitals, I would hope that researchers can be saved from having to deal with unreasonable outside controls on their work. But even now medical researchers, especially when seeking funding, are required to prepare medical and ethical proposals which must be reviewed to assure the appropriateness of the proposed research. This would not change.

FIFTEENTH CONCLUSION:
THE NEED FOR MORAL AND POLITICAL IMAGINATION

The achievement of a just national health care system will call us to new levels of creative moral and political imagination.

I hope it has become clear that the character of modern health care is qualitatively different from the character of earlier health care settings. For this reason the revision of the U.S. health care delivery process is truly a matter of "revisioning," of forming a bold new vision of where we must go and what we must do. To accomplish such imaginative revisioning, all of us need to let go of some of our treasured idols about how medicine, economics, and politics ought to work. We need to become truly free to think new thoughts, hope new hopes, and dream new dreams.[19] To say that we need to let go of some of our cherished convictions does not mean that we should simply abandon these convictions. Instead, in the words of the philosopher Paul Ricoeur, what we need to do is to temporarily suspend our convictions[20] and play with new ideas instead of too quickly rushing to judgment about what is right in terms of health care delivery. It is easy, for instance, to be so convinced that large scale government intervention always messes things up that we never give ourselves the freedom to consider what single payer systems have actually accomplished. It is also easy to be so reflexively in favor of large scale government intervention that we never really consider the problems of such intervention. I know that in writing this book I may very well have been guilty of some of these overly quick judgments, but I have tried—as I think we all must try—to engage both myself and the readers in a true process of imaginative revisioning. To give more emphasis to this theme of imagination, it is hard not to call to mind the words of two of the prophets, first Joel with his hope that sons and daughters will prophesy, that young people will see visions and old people will dream dreams (Jl 3:1–2), and second Habakkuk who said, "The vision has its time, it presses on to its fulfillment. If it delays, wait for it, it will surely come, it will not disappoint" (Hab 2:3). Complete health care reform may well take time, but the vision will indeed come.

To close, I only want to underline something I said near the beginning of the book: modern health care has brought about some truly wonderful accomplishments, and there are many truly wonderful health care professionals in our country who are deeply committed to bringing very high quality service to people who need their care. The health care system has evolved in some complex ways and is clearly in need of change. But this should not obscure the wonder of what has been accomplished or the goodness of the many who bring health care to us. I know that my own outline of key conclusions in this chapter may not offer a perfect set of answers. I hope that I have at least asked the right questions and moved the dialogue further along toward the day when Habakkuk's vision will be true in the field of health care delivery.

POSTSCRIPT

During the weeks in which this book was in the hands of Paulist Press for final editing, typesetting, etc., the most important development in the field of U.S. health care reform was the election of Bill Clinton as president of the United States. As this postscript is written in mid-November of 1992, President-elect Clinton has not yet made any specific legislative proposals on health care reform, so it is uncertain exactly what he will propose. However, from his campaign speeches, it is clear that health care reform will be a high priority for Mr. Clinton. Similarly the general character of Clinton's approach to health care reform is clear from his campaign,[1] even though there was some fluctuation on specific health reform issues as the campaign unfolded. Perhaps the most important single feature of the Clinton approach to health care reform is his commitment to universal access to health care for all Americans, with this access to be provided through a mix of public funding and private, employment-based funding.

Early in the campaign, Clinton tended to argue in favor of a "play or pay" approach to health care reform, i.e. a system in which employers would be required either to provide their employees with health care coverage or be taxed so that the employees could be covered by tax supported plans. More recently, to avoid the possibility of establishing new taxes and larger public programs, Clinton appears to have moved to a "play only" model which will mandate all employers to cover their employees. With either a "play or pay" approach or a "play only" approach, Mr. Clinton is opting for employment-based coverage of working people.

For the unemployed poor who cannot afford to purchase health insurance, Mr. Clinton is clear in his commitment to universal access. But it is unclear whether he favors a single reformed public insurance program or an approach which funds the access of the poor to a variety of state and local coverage settings. The first of these options could either retain both Medicare and Medicaid or it could follow the Pepper Commission's suggestion that the existing multiple public programs (Medicare and Medicaid) be fused into one unified and coherent public insurance program. The second option (public sponsored access to a variety of coverage options in different localities) is based on the recommendations of the Jackson Hole Group, an informal group of health care professionals and business leaders, whose position is supported by the Conservative Democratic Caucus.[2]

In terms of cost containment, Mr. Clinton seems interested in two key methods to help reduce increasing health care costs. One of these methods, most often described as "managed competition," believes that much market-driven cutting of costs can be achieved by enlightened health consumers, both companies and individuals, who can be helped to choose the most cost effective health care plans they can buy. If this managed competition is linked with careful legislation on issues such as a uniform approach to claims processing, Mr. Clinton argues that a good deal of money can be saved. The Clinton approach to managed competition is quite similar to Alain Enthoven's Consumer Choice Program for health care reform which we discussed in Chapter 2. There may be some significant savings available through managed competition, but even some of its proponents acknowledge that it probably cannot work in some health care settings such as sparsely populated areas.[3]

Mr. Clinton's second method of health care cost containment is public regulation of costs through a variety of measures including insurance reform and the establishment of a national health standards board. This board would establish an annual cap on health care spending increases based on growth in the Gross National Product. Such a national cap would be administered through the states. Much work needs to be done to investigate the concept of a national cap on health care expenditures, and it may well be that the Canadian experience with global budgeting for health care (with its pros and cons) will be an important lesson if the U.S. moves to national limits on health care spending.

Besides the elements in the Clinton approach which I have just listed, he has also touched on many other health care reform themes: preventive care, integrated delivery networks, malpractice reform, standardized insurance benefit packages, administrative savings, protection of confidentiality, etc. The early chapters in this book have described many of the basic building blocks which Clinton has used to assemble his program.

I am hesitant to offer too much assessment since President-elect Clinton has not yet made a formal health reform proposal. But in a preliminary assessment of Clinton's campaign positions on health care reform, I offer the following four comments. First, many of the approaches he has suggested have worked well in some of our states or in other countries of the world. Other elements in his approach have not yet been tried, but may also have high potential for good. Thus it is hard not to wish Mr. Clinton the very best in what he hopes to do, especially in terms of the goal of universal access.

Second, from the viewpoint of social justice, I am still troubled by the fact that Mr. Clinton seems to favor a two-tiered health delivery program, with one tier for the employed and the rich who do not work, and a second tier for the poor, who would be covered either by a national program or by local public sponsors. My worries about such an approach are twofold. As an ethicist, my first concern is that the use of a separate financing system for coverage for the poor will leave the poor with a less than adequate standard of health care, meaning that we may not be a truly just society in which all persons have access to a truly reasonable standard of health care. My second more pragmatic worry is that a two-tiered program will be plagued by inefficiencies, thus failing to cut costs and end the current chaos in health care delivery, a chaos which often hurts not only the poor but also the middle class and the rich. While I am open to any health care reform which brings about the human good, I think it is critical that we focus our first attention on how to bring about a truly just health care system. If we begin by deciding what sort of economic philosophy we must use to deliver health care, and then see what health care reform is possible within that economic philosophy, we may not be opening ourselves to a large enough vision of health care justice. And we may not even choose the plan with the highest potential to reduce costs.

Third, I question whether managed competition can truly lead to a more efficient and cost-effective health care system. Do consumers really know what they need or do not need in the field of health care services? In the current, profit-oriented climate of the U.S. insurance industry, can private health insurers, even with many more regulations, be both cost-effective and meet the true health needs of all citizens? For me, it remains hard not to think that a unitary program of health care financing may have the best chance to be both efficient and just in the delivery of health care to all. It might also be important to note that, if the level of coverage provided by such a program is humanly adequate, additional private services may be offered to those who can afford them.

Fourth, I do not think Mr. Clinton's program can be successful unless it establishes a comprehensive national dialogue on what people really need and do not need in the field of health services. For centuries, Roman Catholicism has taught that not every life-prolonging medical intervention is morally required. My view is that this Catholic insight needs to be part of the grounding of an in-depth national dialogue about which health care interventions are truly necessary in a just society. On a related issue, the Bush administration recently ruled that the Oregon Basic Health Services plan is in violation of the Americans With Disabilities Act. Granting that there may be some specific problems with the Oregon plan, I think that this plan was asking a key question about what we must do in the field of health care and what we need not do. In the long run, I do not see how health care reform can succeed unless we ask these deeper questions, and unless we come to an attitude of religious conversion about the meaning of life and death, to a vision which gives us the freedom to let go of life when such letting go is morally appropriate. This question of religious conversion may go beyond the scope of political policy, but it remains a pivotal question if we are going to have a just health care system.

In reflecting on the literary genre of these comments on President-elect Clinton and health care reform, I am reminded of the title of Sören Kierkegaard's *Concluding Unscientific Postscript*.[4] My comments are unscientific because it remains to be seen exactly what Mr. Clinton will propose. My hope for his goal of universal access is genuine. The concerns I have expressed are offered in a spirit of support. They are based on the convictions which I have developed from the entire process of writing this book.

NOTES

NOTES TO INTRODUCTION

[1]George D. Lundberg, "National Health Care Reform: An Aura of Inevitability Is Upon Us," *JAMA* 265 (1991), pp. 2566–2567.

[2]Cf. David Blumenthal, "The Timing and Course of Health Care Reform," *NEJM* 325 (1991), pp. 198–200.

[3]Robert J. Blendon, *et al.*, "Satisfaction With Health Systems in Ten Nations," *Health Affairs* 9 (1990), p. 188.

[4]I refer especially to the notion of proportionality as found in the CDF's *Declaration on Euthanasia* issued on May 5, 1980. In *Origins* 10 (1980), pp. 154–157. This will be discussed in detail in Chapter 4.

[5]NCCB, "Economic Justice For All: Catholic Social Teaching and the U.S. Economy" (Nov. 13, 1986), no. 52. In *Origins* 16 (1986), p. 418.

[6]Philip S. Keane, *Christian Ethics and Imagination* (New York: Paulist Press, 1984).

NOTES TO CHAPTER 1

[1]This figure is cited in Rosemary Kern and Jack Bresch, *Systematic Health Care Reform: Is It Time?* (St. Louis: CHA, 1990), p. 2. Steffie Woolhandler puts the number between 31 and 37 million in the Annual Report of the HCHP (Brookline, Massachusetts, 1990), p. 23.

[2]Emily Friedman, "The Uninsured: From Dilemma to Crisis," *JAMA* 265 (1991), p. 2491.

[3]*Ibid.*, p. 2492.

[4]On February 6, 1992, the Centers for Disease Control reported that the infant mortality rate had reached its lowest point ever: 9.8 first year deaths per 100,000 live births. But this rate is still disturbingly higher than the rate in many other developed countries, and almost twice as high as the infant mortality rate in Japan. The *1992 Britannica Book of the Year* puts the U.S. in 18th lowest place in terms of

its infant mortality rate (Chicago: Encyclopedia Britannica, Inc., 1992, p. 251). For some of the earlier statistics, cf. Charles J. Dougherty, *American Health Care: Realities, Rights, and Reforms* (New York: Oxford University Press, 1988), pp. 3–4.

[5]According to the 1990 Annual Report of the HCHP, life expectancy in the U.S. is 75.6 years compared with 79.2 years for Canada, 76.3 years for Great Britain, 77.2 years in Germany, 77.7 years in Sweden, and 79.3 years in Japan (Cambridge: HCHP, 1990), pp. 4–5.

[6]Friedman, *op. cit.*, p. 2491.

[7]*Ibid.*

[8]Dougherty, *op. cit.*, pp. 4–8.

[9]*Ibid.*, p. 6.

[10]Friedman, *op. cit.*, p. 2491.

[11]Larry R. Churchill, *Rationing Health Care in America: Principles and Perceptions of Justice* (Notre Dame: University of Notre Dame Press, 1987), p. 11. Dougherty, *op. cit.*, p. 9.

[12]Dougherty, *op. cit.*, p. 9.

[13]I say this with two points in mind, first that Medicare does cover virtually everyone over 65, and second that its administrative costs, while high, are less than those for Medicaid or private insurance. David Himmelstein and Steffie Woolhandler, "A National Health Program for the United States: A Physicians' Proposal," *NEJM* 320 (1989), p. 103, report the Medicare administrative cost to be only 2–3% as against 8% for the 1,500 private health insurance carriers in the U.S.

[14]Friedman, *op. cit.*, p. 2492.

[15]On physician refusal to accept Medicaid patients cf. Dougherty, *op. cit.*, pp. 10–11; on the high number of foreign educated physicians (up to 97%) in some hospitals with many poor patients, cf. Dougherty, *op. cit.*, p. 15. Without doubt, many foreign educated doctors are excellent physicians, but the points raised by Dougherty retain their significance.

[16]Paul Cotton, "Preexisting Conditions 'Hold Americans Hostage' to Employers and Insurance," *JAMA* 265 (1991), pp. 2451–2453. The insurors' approaches to preexisting conditions raise questions about the future uses of the human genome project, a congressionally funded study of human gene structures which may give insurors, prospective employers, etc., a great deal of knowledge about the future health status of persons they are considering whether to insure or employ.

[17]On the European attitude toward health insurance, cf. B.L. Kirkman-Liff, "Health Insurance Values and Implementation in the

Netherlands and the Federal Republic of Germany: An Alternative Path to Universal Coverage," *JAMA* 265 (1991), pp. 2496–2502.

[18]One aspect of my caution about the malpractice as a cost factor is this: If it is true that many tests, etc., are sources of extra income for the doctors who request them and the laboratories who perform them, will these tests (which are money makers) stop simply because the fear of lawsuit lessens?

[19]On the attitudes toward death in earlier centuries, cf. Phillipè Aries, "Death Inside Out," in *Death Inside Out* (New York: Harper & Row, 1974), pp. 9–25.

[20]Bruce Hilton, *First Do No Harm: Wrestling with the New Medicine's Life and Death Dilemmas* (Nashville: Abingdon Press, 1991), p. 146.

[21]For the three diseases measles, diptheria, and polio, the U.S. has an average of 70% of its one year olds fully immunized. This percentage is lower than any of the other five countries studied in the recent Harris Survey. Sweden has 97% of its children fully immunized and Canada 85%. For a listing of the UNICEF data on the immunization of children in the countries studied in the Harris Survey, cf. Annual Report of the HCHP (Brookline, 1990), p. 6.

[22]Reported by Howard French in the *New York Times*, February 19, 1989.

[23]Loring Pratt, M.D., "Indigent Patient Care—Then and Now," *Archives of Otolaryngology—Head & Neck Surgery* 117 (1991), pp. 484–485.

[24]Friedman, *op. cit.*, pp. 2493–2494. In reflecting on these figures for uncompensated care, it is hard not to wonder about the effect of laws such as the recent Minnesota law which taxes health care providers in order to cover health care costs.

[25]St. Louis: CHA, 1989.

[26]For an excellent example on how costs continue to be shared in a truly communal fashion, cf. B.L. Kirkman-Liff, *op. cit.*, pp. 2496–2502. For an eloquent summary of the problems of cost shifting in the U.S, cf. Robert Moffit, "Cost Shifting: The Shell Game Played by American Hospitals," The *Baltimore Sun* (May 22, 1992), p. 15A.

[27]Included among the many authors who say that we have a secret system of rationing are Daniel Callahan, *What Kind of Life? The Limits of Medical Progress* (New York: Simon & Schuster, 1990), p. 18; Churchill, *op. cit.*, p. 14; Lundberg, *op. cit.*, pp. 2566–2567.

[28]For an overview of many of the ethical issues related to AIDS, cf. Hessel Bouma III *et al.*, *Christian Faith, Health, & Medical Practice* (Grand Rapids: Wm. B. Eerdmans, 1989), pp. 308–342.

[29]Cf. Eli Ginzberg and Miriam Ostow, "Beyond Universal Insurance to Effective Health Care," *JAMA* 265 (1991), p. 2560.

[30]The most commonly cited figure for 1991 is 11.5% (cf. Cleveland, *op. cit.*, p. 6), meaning that 12% is probably a good estimate for 1992. In the material prepared to accompany the Health USA Act of 1991 (cf. Chapter 2, note 18), Senator Kerrey's office puts the 1990 health care spending at 12.2% of the GNP.

[31]This estimate (from the Division of National Cost estimates) is cited in Kern & Bresch, *op. cit.*, p. 2.

[32]The Kaiser GNP projection was reported to me by John D. Golenski, S.J. of the Bioethics Consultation Group of Berkeley, California.

[33]The most recent figure of $1,086 per car is from David J. Andrea of the University of Michigan Transportation Institute (cf. the *Baltimore Sun*, Feb. 6, 1992, p. 11D).

[34]Robert J. Blendon and Jennifer N. Edwards, "Caring for the Uninsured: Choices For Reform," *JAMA* 265 (1991), p. 2565.

[35]Robert J. Blendon, *et al.*, "Satisfaction With Health Systems in Ten Nations," *Health Affairs* 9 (1990), p. 188.

NOTES TO CHAPTER 2

[1]For a summary of the early history of HMOs, cf. Lee Smith, "Kaiser and the 'Desert Doctors': A Way to Cut Medical Costs," in *Medical Care in the United States* (New York: H.H. Wilson, 1978), pp. 171–173; for a description of HMOs, cf. Thomas & Gloria Mayer, *The Health Insurance Alternative: A Guide to Health Maintenance Organizations* (New York: Perigree Books, 1984).

[2]For a good discussion of some of the ethical problems concerning doctors and joint venturing, cf. Ronald M. Green, "Medical Joint Venturing: An Ethical Perspective," *HCR* 20 (1990), pp. 22–26. On some of the Catholic concerns about joint ventures, cf. *Physician-Hospital Joint Ventures: Ethical Issues* (St. Louis: CHA, 1991). Cf. also Elizabeth McMillan, R.S.M., "Joint Ventures: A Risk to the Ministry's Moral Capital?" *Health Progress* 68 (1987), pp. 54–57, 91.

[3]For an account of the repeal of the catastrophic insurance legislation passed at the end of the Reagan years, cf. "Catastrophic Politics," *National Review* 41 (1989), pp. 12–13.

[4]For critiques of the health care reforms proposed early in the Reagan years, cf. Paul Starr, "The Laissez Faire Elixir," *The New Republic* 188 (1983), pp. 19–23, and Thomas Higgins, "Time for a Second Opinion," *Commonweal* 110 (1983), pp. 365–367.

[5]For an explanation of the Heritage Foundation Proposal, cf. Stuart

M. Butler, "A Tax Reform Strategy to Deal with the Uninsured," *JAMA* 265 (1991), pp. 2541–2544.

[6]For a summary of Kennedy/Waxman, cf. Kern & Bresch, *op. cit.*, pp. 8–9.

[7]James S. Todd, Steven V. Seekins, *et al.*, "Health Access America— Strengthening the US Health Care System," *JAMA* 265 (1991), pp. 2503–2506.

[8]Alain Enthoven and Richard Kronick, "A Consumer Choice Health Plan for the 1990's: Universal Health Insurance in a System Designed to Promote Quality and Economy," *NEJM* 320 (1990), pp. 29–37, 94–101.

[9]National Leadership Commission on Health Care, *For the Health of a Nation* (Ann Arbor: Health Administration Press, 1989).

[10]Cleveland, *op. cit.*, p. 7.

[11]HR5300, The Mediplan Act of 1990. Cf. summaries in Cleveland, *op. cit.*, p. 9, and in Kern & Bresch, *op. cit.*, pp. 8–9.

[12]*A Call For Action: Final Report of the Pepper Commission on Comprehensive Health Care* (Washington, D.C.: Government Printing Office 1990). The Comprehensive Health Care For All Americans Act of 1990. HR4253.

[13]John D. Rockefeller IV, "The Pepper Commission Report on Comprehensive Health Care," *NEJM* 323 (1990), p. 1007.

[14]*Ibid.*, p. 1006.

[15]Cleveland, *op. cit.*, p. 9.

[16]Rashi Fein, "The Health Security Partnership: A Federal-State Universal Insurance and Cost Containment Program," *JAMA* 265 (1991), pp. 2555–2558.

[17]*Ibid.*, p. 2556.

[18]The Health USA Act of 1991, July 11, 1991. Explanatory material on this act was provided to me by Senator Kerrey's office.

[19]Figures cited in the main summary of the Kerrey bill. The independent analysis was done by Lewin/ICF.

[20]Reported in the Baltimore *Evening Sun,* January 27, 1992, p. 8.

[21]David Himmelstein, Steffie Woolhandler, *et al.*, "A National Health Program for the United States: A Physicians' Proposal," *NEJM* 320 (1989), pp. 102–108; Kevin Grumbach, Thomas Bodenheimer, *et al.*, "Liberal Benefits, Conservative Spending: The Physicians for a National Health Program Proposal," *JAMA* 265 (1991), pp. 2549–2554.

[22]Himmelstein and Woolhandler, *op. cit.*, p. 103.

[23]*Ibid.*

[24]HR1300. The Universal Health Care Act of 1991. Introduced by

Mr. Russo on March 6, 1991. Information on the legislation supplied to me by Congressman Russo's office.

[25]In its February 1992 series of reports on the Health Care Crisis, ABC Evening News reported substantially the same figures for the administrative cost of health care.

[26]*The St. Louis Post-Dispatch,* September 1, 1991.

[27]Cf. Martin Gilbert, *Churchill: A Life* (New York: Henry Holt and Company, 1991), p. 742.

[28]For a description of the British system, cf. David Allen, "England," in *Comparative Health Systems: Descriptive Analyses of Fourteen National Health Systems* (University Park: The Pennsylvania State University Press, 1984), pp. 197–257.

[29]Robert J. Blendon, *et al.,* "Satisfaction With Health Systems in Ten Nations," *Health Affairs* 9 (1990), p. 188.

[30]For a description of the Canadian System, cf. Gordon H. Hatcher, et. al., "Canada," in *Comparative Health Systems,* pp. 86–132.

[31]Cf. Blendon, *op. cit.*

[32]Robert Evans, Jonothan Lomas *et al.,* "Controlling Health Expenditures: The Canadian Reality," *NEJM* 320 (1989), p. 572.

[33]*Ibid.*

[34]Adam L. Linton, "The Canadian Health Care System: A Canadian Physician's Perspective," *NEJM* 322 (1990), pp. 197–199.

[35]Cf. Patricia Neighmond, "Health Care in Hawaii," Reports on National Public Radio, July 9–11, 1991. Transcripts available from NPR, 2025 M St. NW, Washington, D.C. 20036.

[36]Friedman, *op. cit.,* p. 2494.

[37]For a description of the Minnesota law (with critical questions), cf. Neal R. Pearce, "Taxing Health Care to Finance Health Care," The *Baltimore Sun,* May 18, 1992, p. 9A.

[38]Joseph P. Ditre, "Making It Work In Maine," *Christianity and Crisis* 51 (1991), pp. 271–273.

[39]For an account of the new Vermont law, cf. Fox Butterfield, "Universal Health Care Plan is Goal of Law in Vermont," *The New York Times* (May 12, 1992), p. 12A.

[40]Harvey D. Klevitt, Alan C. Bates, *et al.,* "Prioritization of Health Care Services: A Progress Report by the Oregon Health Services Commission," *Archives of Internal Medicine* 151 (1991), pp. 912–916.

[41]For a description of all the components in the Oregon plan, as well as an overview of the critical evaluations, cf. Elizabeth O'Connor, "Rationing Health Care: Oregon's Basic Health Services Act" (Unpublished Paper Prepared for the Annual Fellows Forum, February 20, 1991).

[42]Klevitt, Bates, *et al., op. cit.,* p. 912.

[43]For criticisms of Oregon on rationing, cf. Robert M. Veatch, "Should Basic Care Get Priority? Doubts About Rationing the Oregon Way," *Kennedy Institute of Ethics Journal* 1 (1991), pp. 187–206; Robert J. Costagna, "State Health Care Rationing Opposed," *Origins* 21 (1991), pp. 265, 267–268 (Statement for the Oregon Catholic Conference); Bishop James Malone, "Oregon's Health Plan: Step Toward Medical Neglect?" *ibid.,* pp. 270–272. For support of Oregon on the rationing issue cf. Sisters of Providence, "Oregon Health Plan Supported," *ibid.,* p. 269.

NOTES TO CHAPTER 3

[1]Karl Rahner, *On the Theology of Death* (New York: Herder & Herder, 1961), pp. 43–44.

[2]For an important modern treatment of the denial of death, cf. Elisabeth Kübler-Ross, *On Death and Dying* (New York: Macmillan, 1969), pp. 34–43.

[3]If one studies all of the addresses of Pope John Paul II during his first visit to the U.S as pope in 1979, I think a clear case can be made that a deep concern about the overly consumerist character of American life was a major integrating theme in all the addresses which the holy father made. Cf. Pope John Paul II, *Pilgrim of Peace: The Homilies and Addresses of His Holiness Pope John Paul II on the Occasion of His Visit to the United States of America* (Washington: USCC, 1979).

[4]Derek Humphry, *Final Exit: The Practicalities of Self-Deliverance and Assisted Suicide for the Dying* (Eugene: The Hemlock Society, 1991).

[5]Daniel Callahan, *op. cit.,* p. 242. Next chapter we shall point out the long-standing Catholic tradition that we are not required to use ordinary means to prolong life. While this tradition is solidly based, it is true that sometimes arguments against prolonging life slip into the death-avoidance outlook which marks many arguments for suicide and euthanasia. Cf. Paul Ramsey, "The Indignity of Death With Dignity," *HCR* 2 (1974), pp. 47–62.

[6]Karl Rahner, "Proving Oneself in Time of Sickness," *TI* 7 (1971), pp. 275–284.

[7]Second Vatican Council, *Constitution on the Sacred Liturgy,* n. 73.

[8]Karl Rahner, "The Concept of Mystery in Catholic Theology," *TI* 4 (1966), pp. 36–73.

[9]NCCB, *The Challenge of Peace: God's Promise and Our Response* (Washington, D.C.: USCC, 1983, n. 298).

[10]For a radical statement of our role as hopers, cf. Karl Rahner, "On the Theology of Hope," *TI* 10, 1973, pp. 242–259.

[11]These words are inspired by Maria Augusta Neal, *A Socio-Theology of Letting Go* (New York: Paulist Press, 1977).

[12]These comments reflect the modern theology of the fundamental and final option. For the final option cf. Ladislaus Boros, *The Mystery of Death* (New York: Herder & Herder, 1965).

[13]In this context I want to mention the obvious importance of actually telling someone that he or she is dying. The Catholic bishops state this as a requirement in the *Ethical and Religious Directives for Catholic Health Facilities* (St. Louis: CHA, 1976), n. 8.

[14]Cf. Karl Rahner, "The Meaning of Frequent Confession of Devotion," *TI* 3 (1965), pp. 177–189.

[15]For a background on eschatological hope and the transformation of this world, cf. Johannes B. Metz, *Theology of the World* (New York: Herder & Herder, 1969).

[16]Ernst Bloch, *Man on His Own* (New York: Herder & Herder, 1970), p. 161.

[17]On this point, cf. Thomas Aquinas, *Summa Theologica*, II-II, q. 64, a. 4 & a. 6.

[18]*Pastoral Constitution on the Church in the Modern World*, n. 27.

[19]In this context, the "seamless garment" metaphor of Cardinal Bernardin has been especially helpful. Cf. Joseph Cardinal Bernardin *et al.*, *Consistent Ethic of Life* (Chicago: Loyola University of Chicago, 1988).

[20]Thomas Aquinas, *Summa Theologica*, I-II, q. 1.

[21]Pope Pius XII, "The Prolongation of Life" (Nov. 24, 1957), in *The Pope Speaks* 4 (1958), pp. 395–396.

[22]For a summary of key writings on the just war after the Gulf war cf. John Langan, "The Just War Theory After The Gulf War," *TS* 53 (1992) pp. 95–112. Among others, Langan quotes Brian Hehir who said in February 1991: "I am not prepared to declare the entire war unjust purely and simply."

[23]For my own earlier writing on the principle of double effect, cf. Philip S. Keane, "The Objective Moral Order: Reflections on Recent Research," *TS* 43 (1982), pp. 260–278.

[24]The bishops' committee's comments on quality of life are in their document "Nutrition and Hydration: Moral and Pastoral Reflections," n. 5, in *Origins* 21 (1992), pp. 708–709. Among Catholic scholars, Richard Sparks suggests that this careful Catholic position might be called a restricted quality of life position, in *To Treat or Not To Treat: Bioethics and the Handicapped Newborn* (New York: Paulist Press, 1988),

pp. 197–199. Interestingly, in his recent commentary on the Pennsylvania bishops' nutrition/hydration statement, Richard McCormick (whom Sparks uses as an example of a restricted quality of life thinker) does not explicitly articulate quality of life as the basis for his position that nutrition/hydration are not always obligatory for the PVS patient (*America* 166, pp. 210–214).

[25]For a modern classic on this theme of praise, cf. Geoffrey Wainwright, *Doxology: The Praise of God in Worship, Doctrine, and Life* (New York: Oxford University Press, 1980).

[26]Cf. Karl Rahner, "Poetry and the Christian," *TI* 4 (1966), pp. 357–367.

[27]James, M. Gustafson. *Ethics in a Theocentric Context,* 2 vols. (Chicago: University of Chicago Press, 1981, 1984).

[28]*Ibid.,* vol. 1, p. 157.

[29]For a fine summary of global warming, etc., cf. Bill McKibben, *The End of Nature* (New York: Random House, 1989).

[30]John Paul II, *Sollicitudo Rei Socialis* (December 30, 1987), n. 26 (Washington, D.C.: USCC).

[31]Among a growing body of sources, cf. Jerrold Tannenbaum and Andrew Rowan, "Rethinking the Morality of Animal Research," *HCR* 15 (1985), pp. 32–43.

[32]Karl Rahner, "Science as a 'Confession,' " *TI* 3 (1965), p. 387.

[33]In some of the world's languages, the very name for physician (Ger. "artzt") makes this point clear.

[34]Karl Rahner, "The Experiment with Man," *TI* 4 (1966), pp. 216–217.

[35]See especially Abraham Joshua Heschel, *I Asked For Wonder: A Spiritual Anthology* (New York: Crossroad, 1984).

NOTES TO CHAPTER 4

[1]Paul Ramsey, *The Patient as Person* (New Haven: Yale University Press, 1970), pp. 134–135, 151, 153, 161–162.

[2]For a recent account of Dr. Trudeau and the work on TB at Saranac Lake, cf. Robert Taylor, *Saranac: America's Magic Mountain* (Boston: Houghton Mifflin, 1986).

[3]For a brief account of the work of Vittorio, Soto, and Banez, cf. Richard A. McCormick and John J. Paris, "The Catholic Tradition on the Use of Nutrition and Fluids," *America* 156 (1987), p. 358. Cardinal De Lugo will be discussed further when we consider the work of Fr. Gerald Kelly.

⁴For a typical summary of the circumstances which were thought to render a treatment extraordinary, cf. Charles J. McFadden, O.S.A., *Medical Ethics* (Philadelphia: F.A. Davis, 1959), pp. 269–292. In the same time period Edwin F. Healy, S.J. argued that an expense of more than $2,000 rendered a medical treatment extraordinary. Cf. Healy, *Medical Ethics* (Chicago: Loyola University Press, 1956), p. 68.

⁵Gerald Kelly, S.J., "The Duty of Using Artificial Means of Preserving Life," *TS* 11 (1950), p. 208. The examples are from Cardinal De Lugo, *De Justitia et Jure,* Disp. 10, n. 30.

⁶Richard A. McCormick, S.J., *How Brave a New World? Dilemmas in Bioethics* (Garden City: Doubleday, 1981), p. 376 (this section written with Robert Veatch). McCormick is drawing from Gerald Kelly, *Medico-Moral Problems* (St. Louis: The Catholic Hospital Association, 1958), p. 129.

⁷CDF, *Declaration on Euthanasia* (May 5, 1980), n. 4, in *Origins* 10 (1980), p. 156.

⁸This quote is from a document entitled "Essential Elements: Durable Power of Attorney Legislation," issued on January 30, 1992, p. 3.

⁹Richard C. Sparks, C.S.P., *To Treat or Not To Treat: Bioethics and the Handicapped Newborn* (Mahwah: Paulist Press, 1988), pp. 155–255.

¹⁰For a very helpful review of contemporary medical moral thinking on DNR orders, cf. Stuart J. Youngner, "Do-Not-Resuscitate Orders: No Longer a Secret but Still a Problem," *HCR* 17 (1987), pp. 24–33.

¹¹For data on the effect of CPR on certain classes of elderly patients, cf. Donald Murphy, *et al.,* "Outcomes of Cardiopulmonary Resuscitation in the Elderly," *AIM* 111 (1989), pp. 199–205; George E. Taffet, *et al.,* "In-Hospital Cardiopulmonary Resuscitation," *JAMA* 260 (1988), pp. 2069–2071.

¹²Some argue that we should distinguish between cardiac arrests during surgery on a no-code patient which are caused by the anesthesia as distinct from cardiac arrests during surgery on a no-code patient which are caused by the patient's underlying condition, with only the former of these two cases calling for resuscitation. For two recent contributions on this difficult subject cf. Robert M. Walker, "DNR in the OR: Resuscitation as an Operative Risk," *JAMA* 266:17 (November 6, 1991), pp. 2407–2412, and Cynthia B. Cohen and Peter J. Cohen, "Do-Not-Resuscitate Orders in the Operating Room," *NEJM* 325:26 (Dec. 26, 1991), pp. 1879–1882.

¹³In the Catholic tradition, the classic example would be the need to go to confession because one is in the state of mortal sin.

¹⁴*Declaration on Euthanasia,* no. 3, in *Origins* 10 (1980), pp. 155–156.

¹⁵When Gerald Kelly wrote about pneumonia in 1950, the question

was whether some vigorous treatments for pneumonia were extraordinary, even if pneumonia were the only disease which might cause death. Kelly took up the problem of a second disease in the context of whether a diabetic dying of cancer needs to continue on insulin. Kelly, "The Duty of Using Artificial Means of Preserving Life," *TS* 11 (1950), pp. 214, 208–209, 215–216. (Ironically in today's context, Kelly finds the discontinuation of artificial feeding in what he calls "terminal coma" to be easier than any of these other cases.) The theme of pneumonia as a second disease not requiring all possible treatments was well established by the time of John F. Dedek's *Contemporary Medical Ethics* (New York: Sheed & Ward, 1975), pp. 144–146.

[16]NCCB Committee for Pro-Life Activities, "Guidelines for Legislation on Life Sustaining Treatment," Nov. 10, 1984. In *Medical Ethics: Sources of Catholic Teaching* (St. Louis: CHA, 1990), p. 325.

[17]Even the very cautious statement recently adopted by the Pennsylvania bishops shows a clear openness to this type of case. Cf. "Nutrition and Hydration: Moral Considerations," *Origins* 21 (1992), p. 547.

[18]For a discussion of the medical facts of the PVS, cf. Ronald Cranford, "The Persistent Vegetative State: The Medical Reality (Getting the Facts Straight)," *HCR* 18 (1988), pp. 27–32.

[19]Main sources describing the position of McCormick and Paris include: Richard A. McCormick and John J. Paris, "The Catholic Tradition on the Use of Nutrition and Fluids," *America* 156 (1987), pp. 356–361; Richard A. McCormick, "Nutrition/Hydration: The New Euthanasia?" in *The Critical Calling: Reflections on Moral Dilemmas Since Vatican II* (Washington: Georgetown University Press, 1989), pp. 369–388; Richard A. McCormick, " 'Moral Considerations': Ill Considered," *America* 166 (1992), pp. 210–214. In the last of these articles McCormick lists the names (and sometimes written sources) for many authors who share his view.

[20]Cf. William E. May, *et al.*, "Feeding and Hydrating the Permanently Unconscious and Other Vulnerable Persons," *Issues in Law and Medicine* 3 (1987), pp. 203–217; Gilbert Meilander, "The Confused, the Voiceless, the Perverse: Shall We Give Them Food and Drink," *ibid.* 2 (1986), pp. 133–148; John R. Connery, "The Ethical Standards for Withholding/Withdrawing Nutrition and Hydration," *ibid.*, pp. 87–97.

[21]An example of a cautiously open episcopal statement can be seen in Cardinal Joseph Bernardin's "Euthanasia: Legal and Ethical Challenges," *Origins* 18 (1988), esp. p. 52. The Texas bishops' statement, "On Withdrawing Artificial Nutrition/Hydration," is in *Origins* 20 (1990), pp. 53–55; The Oregon/Washington bishops' statement is "Liv-

ing and Dying Well," *Origins* 21 (1991), pp. 335–352; The Pennsylvania bishops' statement is "Nutrition and Hydration: Moral Considerations," *Origins* 21 (1992), pp. 543–553. Some of these statements (and some of the articles cited in the previous two notes) take up issues which I am not able to treat here, such as whether a PVS patient can feel any pain, and whether the withdrawal of nutrition/hydration is a permitting or a causing of death.

[22]NCCB Pro-Life Committee, "Nutrition and Hydration: Moral and Pastoral Considerations," *Origins* 21 (1992), pp. 705–712.

[23]I say "normally" because a Catholic hospital would clearly not be obligated to provide euthanasia to a patient who requests it. Similarly, I think that neither hospital nor physician would be obligated to provide manifestly futile treatment to any patient.

[24]*Declaration on Euthanasia*, n. 4, in *Origins* 10 (1980), p. 156.

[25]I refer here to the famous Cruzan decision. For evaluative comments on the decision by several authors, cf. "Cruzan: Clear and Convincing," *HCR* 20 (1991), pp. 5–11.

[26]I say nothing formally wrong, because there could be specific elements in a given piece of advance directive legislation to which Catholic teaching might object. Also, Catholic teaching might well seek to have certain conditions present in advance directive legislation, e.g. a stipulation that a durable power of attorney does not apply to the withdrawal of nutrition/hydration unless the person giving the power explicitly stipulates that the attorney in fact has the power to withdraw nutrition/hydration.

[27]While I found it quite helpful, I thought there was some of this strong autonomy tone in the video *On Your Behalf: Your Right to Refuse or Accept Medical Treatment*. CAREsource Program Development, Inc., 505 Seattle Tower, 1218 Third Ave., Seattle, WA 98101.

[28]*Declaration on Euthanasia*, n. 4, in *Origins* 10 (1980), p. 156.

[29]For an example of the futility literature (with references), cf. Daniel Callahan, "Medical Futility/Medical Necessity: The Problem Without a Name," *HCR* 21 (1991), pp. 30–35.

[30]In other words, at least until the categories can be more carefully defined, I am more at peace with a quantitative notion of futility than with a qualitative notion. Cf. Lawrence Schneiderma, Nancy Jecker, and Albert Jonsen, "Medical Futility: Its Meaning and Ethical Implications," *AIM* 112 (1990), pp. 949–954.

[31]For Ramsey's position, cf. Paul Ramsey, *The Patient as Person* (cf. note 1 above), pp. 144–164. For Callahan, cf. "Aid-In-Dying," *Commonweal* 118 (1991), pp. 476–480, and "When Self-Determination Runs

Amok," *HCR* 22 (1992), pp. 52–55; for John Paris, cf. "Active Euthanasia," *TS* 53 (1992), pp. 113–126; for a report on the Netherlands, cf. Maurice A.M. de Wachter, "Euthanasia in the Netherlands," *HCR* 22 (1992), pp. 30–33.

[32]Cf. the statement of the bishops of Washington, "Initiative 119: The Real Choice," *Origins* 21 (1991), p. 302.

[33]Cf. Chapter 3, note 5.

[34]Richard McCormick has recently argued this point very well and asserted that the implementation of the Catholic ethic might actually help reduce the push for euthanasia. Cf. Richard A. McCormick, "Biomedical Problems in the Nineties," *New Catholic World* 234 (1991), pp. 197–201; Archbishop Thomas Murphy, speaking for the bishops of Oregon and Washington, made a very favorable use of Fr. McCormick's argument; cf. *Origins* 21 (1991), p. 300.

[35]I will discuss the relation of church teaching on euthanasia and similar issues to the question of public policy for health reform in Chapter 7.

[36]I understand the real fear which some have that health reform will lead to individual treatment decisions being made on the basis of the cost of a treatment. I think steps like those I have just mentioned can prevent this fear from becoming a reality. Later we will take up the ethics of health care rationing, but there the focus will be on how to treat whole classes of patients, not on setting an economic criterion for individual treatment decisions.

NOTES TO CHAPTER 5

[1]Probably the classic example of a pre-Vatican II Catholic thinker whose roots are almost completely philosophical is Msgr. John A. Ryan whom we will be considering later. In particular it is fascinating to compare Ryan's *Distributive Justice* (New York: Macmillan, 1916) with the Protestant scholar Walter Rauschenbusch's *A Theology for the Social Gospel* (Nashville: Abingdon Press, 1917). Written in the same time period and relying on the same economists, Rauschenbusch is replete with scripture quotes while Ryan has only a handful of scripture quotes in five hundred pages.

[2]For the importance of the radical monotheism theme, cf. H. Richard Niebuhr, *Radical Monotheism and Western Culture* (New York: Harper & Row, 1970).

[3]For an excellent presentation of this trinitarian theology, focusing

especially on the relation between God's life (the immanent Trinity) and our communal life (the economic Trinity), cf. Karl Rahner, *The Trinity* (New York: Herder & Herder, 1970), esp. p. 22.

[4]Karl Rahner, "Atheism and Implicit Christianity," *TI* 9 (1972), pp. 145–164.

[5]Karl Rahner, "The Concept of Mystery in Catholic Theology," *TI* 4 (1966), pp. 36–73.

[6]Karl Rahner, "The Question of the Future," *TI* 12 (1974), p. 185. Also crucially important in this context is Rahner's "On the Theology of Hope," *TI* 10 (1973), pp. 242–259.

[7]Pius XII, *Mystici Corporis* (June 29, 1943), n. 12.

[8]Second Vatican Council, *Dogmatic Constitution on the Church* (*Lumen Gentium*), chapter 2.

[9]*The Rule of St. Benedict* (Collegeville, 1980), pp. 274–275 (chapter 61).

[10]For the historical development of hospitals (and earlier institutions such as *valetudinaria, infirmatoria, leprosaria,* and *hotels dieu*), cf. W. Douglas Piercey and Harold Scarborough, "Major Medical Institutions: Hospitals," in *Encyclopaedia Britannica* 23 (15th ed.; Chicago, 1989), pp. 914–915, and Kenneth J. Williams, "Hospitals," in *Encyclopedia of Bioethics* 2 (New York: Macmillan and Free Press, 1978), pp. 677–683.

[11]Often today, when Catholic hospitals revise their mission statements, the revised statements specifically include an advocacy role. Likewise, Catholic health care systems are now likely to include an office for advocacy as well as an office for ethics.

[12]For the place of beauty in Christian ethics, cf. Bernard Häring, "A Morality of Beauty and Glory," in *Free and Faithful in Christ: Moral Theology for Priests and Laity* 2 (New York: Seabury Press, 1979), pp. 102–152.

[13]In the context of beauty and health care, I want to stress the importance of tasteful religious art and symbols as part of the health care setting. An awareness of the many diverse religious traditions of patients led some Catholic hospitals into a period of deemphasizing religious art and symbols. Happily, many Catholic health care institutions are today rediscovering the importance of art and religious symbols as statements of the deeper wholeness which must be part of a sound approach to health care delivery.

[14]For Troeltsch's comparison of churches and sects, cf. Ernst Troeltsch, *The Social Teaching of the Christian Churches* 1 (New York: Harper & Row, 1960), pp. 331–343.

[15]Cf. Troeltsch's comments on Leo Tolstoy, *ibid.* 2, pp. 728–729.

[16]I refer to the famous *Bishops' Program of Social Reconstruction* of February 11, 1919. In *American Catholic Thought on Social Questions* (Indianapolis: Bobbs-Merrill, 1968), pp. 325–348.

[17]Karl Rahner, "The Unity of Spirit and Matter in the Christian Understanding of Faith," *TI* 6 (1969), p. 168.

[18]Thomas Aquinas, *Summa Theologica*, q. 84, a. 7.

[19]Karl Rahner, "Reflections on the Unity of the Love of Neighbor and the Love of God," *TI* 6 (1969), pp. 231–249.

[20]Martin Luther King, "Nonviolence: The Only Road to Freedom," in *A Testament of Hope: The Essential Writings of Martin Luther King, Jr.* (New York: Harper & Row, 1986), p. 58; cf. Kenneth Smith & Ira Zepp, *The Search for the Beloved Community: The Thinking of Martin Luther King, Jr.* (Valley Forge: Judson Press, 1974).

[21]I think Rahner's best statement of this whole divinization theme is found in his "Christology Within an Evolutionary View of the World," *TI* 5 (1968), esp. p. 183.

[22]The classic twentieth century history of natural law is Odon Lottin, *Le Droit Natural chez Thomas d'Aquin et ses prédécesseurs* (Bruges: Charles Beyart, 1931).

[23]For a summary of the positive Catholic view of government, cf. Heinrich Rommen, *The State in Catholic Thought* (St. Louis: B. Herder, 1945), esp. pp. 282–305.

[24]Reinhold Niebuhr, *The Children of Light and the Children of Darkness: A Vindication of Democracy and a Critique of Its Traditional Defense* (New York: Charles Scribner's, 1944), pp. 144–145.

[25]NCCB, *The Challenge to Peace: God's Promise and Our Response* (Washington: USCC, 1983), nn. 8–9.

[26]John C. Bennett, "Ecumenical Co-operation on Public Issues," *Concilium* 4 (1969), p. 38. For further explanation, cf. Bennett, *Christians and the State* (New York: Charles Scribner's, 1958), pp. 13–23.

[27]For a description of the two realm theory, cf. Martin Luther, "On Secular Authority: To What Extent It Should Be Obeyed," in *Martin Luther: Selections From His Writings* (Garden City: Doubleday & Co., 1961), pp. 368–373.

[28]*Ibid.*, pp. 382–392.

[29]John Calvin, *Institutes of the Christian Religion*, Book 2, Chapter 8, no. 5, Library of Christian Classics Edition (Philadelphia: Westminster Press, 1960), vol. 1, p. 372.

[30]H. Richard Niebuhr, *Christ and Culture* (New York: Harper & Row, 1951), pp. 144–147.

214   *Health Care Reform*

³¹Notre Dame: University of Notre Dame Press, 1981.
³²Notre Dame: University of Notre Dame Press, 1981.
³³Berkeley: University of California Press, 1985.

NOTES TO CHAPTER 6

¹This can even be seen in the U.S. Constitution with its system of checks and balances and its impeachment clause. Checks and balances prevent anyone from having too much power, power which one might well be tempted to use in a sinful manner.

²In my view the *Bishops' Program for Social Reconstruction* (cf. chapter 5, note 16) and many of the bishops' documents which have followed it over the years fall into this "mixed economy pattern."

³*Rerum Novarum,* n. 34.

⁴*Ibid.,* nn. 4, 11–12.

⁵Pius XI, *Quadragesimo Anno,* nn. 45–46, 56–57, and esp. no. 79.

⁶Paul VI, *Populorum Progressio* (March 26, 1967), n. 24.

⁷Pope John Paul II, *Sollicitudo Rei Socialis* (December 30, 1987), n. 21.

⁸*Pacem in Terris* (April 11, 1963), nn. 11–27.

⁹Second Vatican Council, *Declaration on Religious Liberty,* nn. 1–8.

¹⁰Synod of Bishops, Second General Assembly, *Justice in the World* (Nov. 30, 1971), n. 6.

¹¹Cf. Charles M. Murphy, "Action for Justice as Constitutive of the Preaching of the Gospel: What Did the 1971 Synod Mean?" *TS* 44 (1983), pp. 298–311.

¹²Mary Ann Glendon, *Rights Talk: The Impoverishment of Political Discourse* (New York: The Free Press, 1991).

¹³It is difficult to come up with the best way of expressing the idea of health care as a right. Once we grant that it is impossible to assure that everyone will be healthy, the question becomes what standard of services we must make available to help people become and stay healthy. In the Preamble to its Constitution, the World Health Organization speaks of a right to the highest attainable standard of health. In 1944 Franklin D. Roosevelt spoke about the "right to adequate medical care." The AMA in 1969 spoke of the right of every citizen to adequate health care. Charles Fried speaks about a decent, fair standard or a decent minimum. Here I have used the term "basic standard." For reflections on all this, cf. Carleton B. Chapman and John M. Talmadge, "The Evolution of the Right to Health Concept in the United States," in *EM,* esp. pp. 553–554, and

Charles M. Fried, "Equality and Rights in Medical Care," *ibid.*, pp. 580–583.

[14]Cf. Paul Starr, *The Social Transformation of American Medicine* (New York: Basic Books, 1982), pp. 154–162.

[15]For an excellent historical survey, cf. Chapman and Talmadge, *op. cit.*, pp. 554–572.

[16]*Pacem in Terris*, n. 11.

[17]*Laborem Exercens*, n. 19.

[18]NCCB, *Health and Health Care* (Nov. 19, 1981), n. 2, in *Pastoral Letters of the United States Catholic Bishops* 4 (Washington: USCC 1984), p. 469.

[19]For a description of the responsible society, cf. H.D. Wedland, "The Theology of the Responsible Society," in *Christian Social Ethics in a Changing World* (New York: Association Press, 1966), pp. 135–152.

[20]David Gill, ed., *Gathered for Life: Official Report VI Assembly World Council of Churches* (Grand Rapids: Eerdmans, 1983).

[21]For a Catholic overview of the common good, cf. Jacques Maritain, *The Person and the Common Good* (New York: Charles Scribner's, 1947); cf. also Maritain's excellent short summary in his *Man and the State* (Chicago: University of Chicago Press, 1951), pp. 11–12.

[22]For a description of some of the controversies surrounding the common good in the 1940s, cf. Ralph McInerny, "The Primacy of the Common Good," in *The Common Good and U.S. Capitalism*, ed. by Oliver Williams and John Houck (Lanham: University Press of America, 1987), pp. 70–83.

[23]Pope John Paul II, *Centesimus Annus*, n. 13.

[24]Maritain, *Man and the State*, p. 24.

[25]This point is highlighted by Oliver Williams, in "To Enhance the Common Good: An Introduction," in Williams and Houck, *op. cit.*, p. 1.

[26]Curran, "The Common Good and Official Catholic Social Teaching," in Williams and Houck, *op. cit.*, pp. 113–117.

[27]Dennis McCann, "The Good to be Pursued in Common," in Williams and Houck, *op. cit.*, pp. 158–178.

[28]*Centesimus Annus*, n. 47.

[29]Cf. John Cobb and Herman Daly, *For the Common Good: Redirecting the Economy Toward Community, the Environment, and a Sustainable Future* (Boston: Beacon Press, 1989).

[30]Robert Bellah *et al.*, *The Good Society* (New York: Alfred A. Knopf, 1991).

[31]Bellah *et al.*, *Habits of the Heart: Individualism and Commitment in American Life* (Berkeley: University of California Press, 1985).

³²Robert Bellah *et al., The Good Society,* p. 7.

³³*Ibid.,* pp. 270–286.

³⁴For a typical manualist treatment of the three kinds of justice, cf. John McHugh and Charles Callan, *Moral Theology: A Complete Course* (London: B. Herder, 1958), vol. 2, pp. 36–38.

³⁵For a survey of many of the labor issues in health care, cf. Adam Maida, ed., *Issues in the Labor/Management Dialogue: Church Perspectives* (St. Louis: CHA, 1982).

³⁶Robert Bellah *et al., The Good Society,* pp. 70–72.

³⁷Cf., e.g., Alan Geyer and Barbara Green, *Lines in the Sand: Justice and the Gulf War* (Westminster: John Knox, 1992).

³⁸New York: Macmillan, 1916.

³⁹*Ibid.,* pp. 212–222.

⁴⁰For an excellent statement of the case for affirmative action, cf. Daniel C. Maguire, *A New American Justice: Ending the White Male Monopolies* (Garden City: Doubleday, 1980), esp. pp. 27–51.

⁴¹NCCB, *Economic Justice for All: Catholic Social Teaching and the U.S. Economy* (Nov. 13, 1986) n. 52, in *Origins* 16:24 (1986), p. 418.

⁴²Charles E. Curran, "The Common Good and Official Catholic Social Teaching," in Williams and Houck, *op. cit.,* pp. 124–125.

⁴³Cf. David Hollenbach, *Claims in Conflict: Retrieving and Renewing the Catholic Human Rights Tradition* (New York: Paulist Press, 1979), pp. 54–56.

⁴⁴In the context of overemphasizing commutative justice, it is hard not to think of the image (popular in some quarters) of the doctor as baker, selling his goods to whoever can pay the price. Cf. Robert M. Sade, "Medical Care as a Right: A Refutation," in *EM,* pp. 573–576.

⁴⁵Cambridge: Harvard University Press, 1971, esp. p. 83.

⁴⁶Gene Outka, "Social Justice and Equal Access to Health Care," in *EM,* pp. 584–592.

⁴⁷Daniel Callahan, *Setting Limits: Medical Goals in an Aging Society* (New York: Simon & Schuster, 1987); *With Justice For All? The Ethics of Health Care Rationing* (St. Louis: CHA, 1991).

⁴⁸While Ramsey made this line famous, it actually comes from David Sanders and Jesse Dukeminier, Jr., "Medical Advance and Legal Lag: Hemodialysis and Kidney Transplantation," in *EM,* p. 610.

⁴⁹Outka, *op. cit.,* p. 588.

⁵⁰*Ibid.,* p. 590.

⁵¹Cf. note 47 above.

⁵²This was the point of Stephen G. Post's paper "Good Parents, Agape, and Ordo Amoris," which was presented at the January 1992 meeting of the Society of Christian Ethics.

[53]It is interesting to note that the contemporary concern about the quality of education in the U.S. began at almost the same time that the cost and complexity of health care began to become an issue of concern. Consider, for instance, the publication date of Charles E. Silberman's famous *Crisis in the Classroom: The Remaking of American Education* (New York: Random House, 1970).

[54]CHA, *With Justice For All?* p. 22, n. 19.

[55]Cf. Chapter 1, note 25.

[56]Cf. note 47 above.

[57]*Quadragesimo Anno*, n. 79.

[58]In nn. 99–101 of their 1986 pastoral letter *Economic Justice for All*, the Catholic bishops of the United States describe the principle of subsidiarity especially in terms of pluralism. In *Origins* 16 (1986), p. 422.

[59]*Mater et Magistra*, nn. 116–121; *Laborem Exercens*, n. 14.

[60]Cf. William E. Simon and Michael Novak, "Pope's Encyclical Advances Liberty, Prosperity," *National Catholic Reporter* (May 24, 1991), p. 32.

NOTES TO CHAPTER 7

[1]For an example of a great twentieth century theologian struggling with the distinction between what one does as an official and as a private person, cf. Emil Brunner, *The Divine Imperative* (Philadelphia: Westminster Press, 1947 [orig. 1932]), esp. pp. 220–233. Brunner does state that both official and private actions must come from love, but still there is often a difference between the actions themselves.

[2]Martin Luther, "On Secular Authority: To What Extent It Should Be Obeyed," in *Martin Luther: Selections from His Writings* (Garden City: Doubleday & Co., 1961), pp. 363–402.

[3]Cf. Thomas Sanders, *Protestant Concepts of Church and State* (Garden City: Doubleday, 1965), pp. 70–73.

[4]Cf. H. Richard Niebuhr, *Christ and Culture* (New York: Harper and Row, 1951), pp. 217–218.

[5]One of the interesting aspects of the events leading to the establishment of prohibition is the link between the anti-women suffrage and anti-prohibition forces; cf. Eleanor Flexnor, *Century of Struggle: The Women's Rights Movement in the United States* (Cambridge: Harvard University Press, 1975), pp. 306–309.

[6]For an articulate critique of the "my religion is one thing, but my

politics are separate" outlook, cf. Cardinal John O'Connor, "Abortion: Questions and Answers," *Origins* 20 (1990), p. 105.

[7]The classic modern summary of the Thomistic approach is found in John Courtney Murray's works, especially in *We Hold These Truths: Catholic Reflections on the American Proposition* (Garden City: Doubleday, 1964). Also very helpful are Charles E. Curran, "Civil Law and Christian Morality: Abortion and the Churches," in *Ongoing Revision Studies in Moral Theology* (Notre Dame: Fides Press, 1975), pp. 107–143; Christopher F. Mooney, *Public Virtue: Law and the Social Character of Religion* (Notre Dame: University of Notre Dame Press, 1986); Thomas R. Ulshafer, S.S., "On the Morality of Legislative Compromise: Some Historical Underpinnings," *Linacre Quarterly* 59 (1992), pp. 10–26.

[8]Heinrich Rommen, *The State in Catholic Thought* (St. Louis: B. Herder, 1945), esp. pp. 248–268, 571.

[9]For a summary of Thomas Aquinas on these questions, cf. Murray, *op. cit.*, pp. 164–165.

[10]For Pope Pius XII's views, cf. his "Crime and Punishment," in *Contemporary Punishment: Views, Explanations and Justifications* (Notre Dame: University of Notre Dame Press, 1972), pp. 59–72.

[11]NCCB, "Statement on Capital Punishment," *Origins* 10 (1980), pp. 373–377.

[12]For a summary of some of the post-Roe vs. Wade comments on abortion and public policy cf. Richard A. McCormick, *Notes on Moral Theology 1965–1980* (Lanham: University Press of America, 1981), pp. 479–493. Also interesting in this context is the famous address of Gov. Mario Cuomo at Notre Dame in 1984 entitled "Religious Belief and Public Morality," in *Origins* 14 (1984–85), pp. 234–240. In this address, Gov. Cuomo seems to have captured at least some of the traditional Catholic nuances about morality and public policy. But it may well be that some of his more recent statements, at least if reported correctly in the press, have lost this careful nuancing. Later in the text we will discuss the statements of Archbishop John R. Quinn (in *Origins* 14 [1984], pp. 221–222) and Cardinal John O'Connor (*op. cit.*, p. 106).

[13]Reinhold Niebuhr, *The Children of Light and the Children of Darkness: A Vindication of Democracy and a Critique of Its Traditional Defense* (New York: Charles Scribner's, 1994), pp. 144–145. In *We Hold These Truths*, p. 164, John Courtney Murray takes a position somewhat similar to Niebuhr's.

[14]For a manual explanation of the traditional principles on cooperation in evil, cf. John McHugh and Charles Callan, *Moral Theology: A Complete Course* (London: B. Herder, 1958), vol. 1, pp. 603–628. These authors first divide material cooperation into immediate and

mediate material cooperation, with immediate cooperation (e.g. actual assistance in an abortion as distinct from prepping or aftercare) being so close to the action that it can never be justified. With this in mind only mediate material cooperation (which can be either proximate or remote) can be morally justified on the basis of a sufficient reason.

[15]For discussion of these kinds of cases, cf. Charles McFadden, *Medical Ethics* (Philadelphia: F.A. Davis, 1951), pp. 304–322; Benedict Ashley and Kevin O'Rourke, *Health Care Ethics: A Theological Analysis* (St. Louis: CHA, 1989, pp. 188–190, 224; Catholic Bishops of the State of Connecticut, "Catholic Health Personnel and Abortion," *Origins* 4 (1974–75), pp. 171–174.

[16]Cf. Charles E. Curran, "Cooperation in a Pluralistic Society," in *Ongoing Revision*, pp. 210–228.

[17]CDF, *Instruction on Human Life in Its Origin and on the Dignity of Procreation*, Part III, February 22, 1987 (in Thomas Shannon and Lisa Cahill, *Religion and Artificial Reproduction* [New York: Crossroad, 1988], p. 169), appears to reject Curran's approach.

[18]On the subject of Catholic dioceses joining in United Way campaigns, cf. "A Pastoral Letter on Moral Decision Making," by retired Archbishop Raymond G. Hunthausen of Seattle. The text of the letter appeared in the *Catholic Northwest Progress* on October 1, 1976.

[19]NCCB Statement on Tubal Ligation, *Origins* 10 (1980–81), p. 175; CDF, "Sterilization in Catholic Hospitals" (March 13, 1975), in *Medical Ethics: Sources of Catholic Teaching* (St. Louis: CHA, 1989), pp. 293–294.

[20]I think, for example, of England where moves for health care reform began early in the twentieth century, but where it was not until the late 1940s that the current delivery system was put into place.

[21]The figure of 9.8 million more persons who could buy health insurance if it were fully deductible was developed by the non-partisan group, Health Care Solutions for America (reported by Tom Bowman in the *Baltimore Sun*, February 14, 1992, p. 3A).

[22]President Bush specifically endorsed such an approach to welfare mothers and infants in his news conference on April 10, 1992. I realize that this issue is technically speaking a welfare reform issue rather than a health care justice issue. But I still think we must consider the health care implications for the children who are affected by the proposal.

[23]Washington: USCC, 1975, n. 12.

[24]Cardinal O'Connor, *op. cit.,* p. 103.

[25]All the publicity surrounding basketball star Magic Johnson has moved the debate between the "safe sex" advocates and the abstinence advocates more clearly into the foreground. It is in this context that I

think the abstinence position may well gain more adherents, though the tension between the two positions will continue.

[26]One of the most interesting sociological studies of the question of what kind of abortion legislation may be sociologically feasible in the U.S. is Kristin Luker's *Abortion and the Politics of Motherhood* (Berkeley: University of California Press, 1984).

[27]For the statements of Archbishop Quinn and Cardinal O'Connor, cf. note 12 above. A complete theological treatment of abortion, both from the moral viewpoint and from the public policy viewpoint, would require the consideration of many issues which are beyond the scope of this book. Here the purpose is to present the clear Catholic teaching on abortion and public policy so as to show the possible implications of this teaching for health care reform.

[28]*Ibid.*, p. 106.

[29]In the past few paragraphs I have focused on the relation between abortion and health care reform legislation because of the great importance of the issues involved. While we will not discuss issues such as the relation of health care reform to AIDS education, the same basic principles should be applied.

NOTES TO CHAPTER 8

[1]Most of the assertions made in this chapter will be based on sources developed and cited in the earlier chapters. Hence notes will occur in this chapter only when there are references to new sources or when it seems especially helpful to refer back to material discussed in previous parts of the book.

[2]Cf. Chapter 2, note 29.

[3]Cf. Chapter 2, note 18.

[4]Reinhold Niebuhr, *Moral Man and Immoral Society* (New York: Charles Scribner's, 1932), esp. pp. xi–xii.

[5]Niebuhr's Augustinian turn is seen most clearly in his *The Nature and Destiny of Man* (New York: Charles Scribner's, 1941, 1943), esp. vol. 1, pp. 152–159, and vol. 2, pp. 272–274.

[6]Reinhold Niebuhr, *Man's Nature and His Communities* (New York: Charles Scribner's, 1965), p. 22.

[7]Cf. Chapter 2, note 29.

[8]Marty Russo, "Single Payer System Guarantees Health Care for Less," *The Christian Science Monitor* (September 10, 1991), p. 1.

[9]For an account of the European successes in covering health care

needs, cf. Mark Maremont, *et al.*, "Can Europe Help Cure America's Health Care Mess?" *Business Week* (March 9, 1992), pp. 52–54.

[10]For an account of the struggle to unify the armed services under one cabinet secretary, cf. Clark Clifford, *Counsel to the President* (New York: Random House, 1991), pp. 146–174.

[11]In this context it should be noted that in his recent encyclical *Centesimus Annus*, nn. 32 and 35, Pope John Paul II speaks positively about the role of business, of profit, competition, etc.

[12]*Setting Relationships Aright: Shaping CHA's Proposal For Systematic Health Care Reform* (St. Louis: CHA, 1991), p. 31 of section entitled "Means of Achieving Delivery Reform."

[13]*Ibid.*, p. 22.

[14]Louis Harris and Associates, *Comparing Health Systems: An International Survey of Consumer Satisfaction* (Cambridge: HCHP, 1990), p. 1. Canada's citizens were more satisfied with their health system than the citizens of any other nation in the survey.

[15]For a compendium of articles on conversion, including seminal works by Bernard Lonergan, Reinhold Niebuhr, Karl Barth, and Karl Rahner, cf. Walter Conn, ed., *Conversion: Perspectives on Personal and Social Transformation* (Staten Island: Alba House, 1978).

[16]The theme of age and the critique of Callahan was touched upon by several papers (and follow-up discussions of the papers) at the January 1992 annual meeting of the Society of Christian Ethics, including Per Andersen's "On the Ragged Edge of Medical Progress: Daniel Callahan and the Question of Limits," and Barbara Andolsen's "Justice, Gender, and the Frail Elderly: Reexamining an Ethic of Care." For Callahan's own comments on age, cf. his *Setting Limits* (cited in chapter 6, n. 47), pp. 164–174.

[17]One small comparison: Bangladesh's figure for life expectancy for both males and females is 56. The infant mortality rate is 98 per 1,000 births. There is one doctor for each 6,000 people, and one hospital bed for each 300 people. In the U.S. life expectancy is 72 for white men and 79 for white women. The infant mortality rate is 9.1 per 1,000 births. There is one physician for each 400 persons and one hospital bed for each 200 persons. And, as mentioned earlier, the U.S. figures are often worse than figures for Canada and the western European countries. The figures are from the *1992 Britannica Book of the Year* (Chicago: Encyclopaedia Britannica, Inc.), pp. 550–551, 725, 728.

[18]These comments on sovereignty are drawn from a paper presented by Rev. J. Brian Hehir at the *Journal of Religious Ethics Forum*

which preceded the 1992 Annual Meeting of the Society of Christian Ethics.

[19]Cf. Philip S. Keane, *Christian Ethics and Imagination* (New York: Paulist Press, 1984).

[20]A helpful example of Ricoeur's thinking along these lines is "The Metaphorical Process as Cognition, Imagination, and Feeling," *Critical Inquiry* 5 (1978), pp. 143–159.

NOTES TO POSTSCRIPT

[1]For a summary in Clinton's own words, cf. Bill Clinton, "The Clinton Health Care Plan," *NEJM* 327:11 (September 10, 1992), pp. 804–807.

[2]For a summary of the Jackson Hole Group's approach, cf. Alain C. Enthoven, "Commentary: Measuring the Candidates on Health Care," *ibid.*, pp. 807–809.

[3]Cf. H.E. Simmons, *et al.*, "Comprehensive Health Care Reform and Managed Competition," *NEJM* 327:21 (November 19, 1992), p. 1527.

[4]Sören Kierkegaard, *Concluding Unscientific Postscript to the 'Philosophical Fragments,'* Oxford: Oxford University Press, 1941.

ABBREVIATIONS

AIM	*Annals of Internal Medicine*
CDF	Congregation for the Doctrine of the Faith
CHA	The Catholic Health Association of the United States
EM	*Ethics in Medicine: Historical Perspectives and Contemporary Concerns,* ed. by Stanley Reiser, Arthur Dyck, and William Curran (Cambridge: MIT Press, 1977)
HCHP	Harvard Community Health Plan
HCR	*Hastings Center Report*
JAMA	*Journal of the American Medical Association*
NCCB	National Conference of Catholic Bishops
NEJM	*New England Journal of Medicine*
TI	Karl Rahner, *Theological Investigations,* 20 vols (London: Darton, Longman, & Todd, 1961–1992)
TS	*Theological Studies*
USCC	United States Catholic Conference

INDEX

AIDS 28, 68, 81, 183, 210, 220

Abortion 71–72, 154, 159, 161–62, 164, 167–71, 218–20

Access to health care 40, 128, 135, 138–39, 145, 164–67, 170–71, 184, 186, 191, 195, 198

Administrative cost of health care 48–49, 52, 165, 175–76

Advance directives 93–94, 100

Agape 114

Age and health care 11, 86, 128, 140, 147, 190, 221

American Medical Association 40–41

Americans With Disabilities Act 198

Andolsen, Barbara 221

Animal rights 76–77

Anointing of the Sick 65

Aquinas, Thomas 3, 72, 75, 77, 113, 115, 119, 121, 124, 130, 132, 135, 156, 177, 206, 213, 218

Aristotle 115, 121, 124, 130, 135

Art of the possible 156, 159, 166, 169, 188

Asceticism 66–67, 77

Ashley, Benedict, 219

Athletics 62–63, 121

Augustine 177, 220

Automobile cost and health care 30, 193

Autonomy 84, 92, 94–95, 97, 101, 126, 147, 156–57, 160, 164

Baptism 111

Barth, Karl 221

Basic Health Care For All Americans Act 40

Beauty and health care 110

Bellah, Robert 120, 132, 215–16

Bennett, John C. 117, 213

Bernardin, Joseph 209

Bill of Rights 123

Bishops' Pro-Life Committee 74, 89, 91, 209–10

Blendon, Robert 119, 202, 204

Bloch, Ernst 71, 206

Borglum, Gutzon 81

Bouma, Hessel 201

Brandeis, Louis 46

Bresch, John 199, 201, 203

Brunner, Emil 217

Buckley, William F. 149

Burdens and benefits 13, 84–86, 90–92, 95, 97, 137, 147–48, 189–91

Bush, George 39, 219

Business leaders and health care 30

Calvin, John, and Calvinism 199, 155–156, 213

Canada 31, 50–55, 126–27, 175, 181, 184, 188, 200–01, 204

Canons of Justice 137, 139–43

Cap on national health care expense 196

Capital punishment 158, 218

Capitalism, 124–25, 149

Capitation fee 33, 48

Cardiopulmonary resuscitation 86–87, 96, 208

Care for the dying 80–102

Carter, Jimmy 36

Catastrophic illness 14, 36, 202

Catholic Health Association 24, 140, 147–48, 181, 183, 208, 221

Catholic bishops and right to care 129, 215

Catholic legislators 159, 167, 169–71

Catholic moral tradition 5, 13, 19, 26, 39, 69, 71–72, 80, 82, 84–85, 98–99, 102, 119–120, 125, 129–31, 133, 142–43, 153–54, 156–58, 166–67, 169, 172, 178–79, 208, 210

Catholic philosophy 115–121

Catholic social teaching 122, 124–25, 177, 216

Catholicism and health care reform 164–172

Centesimus Annus 130–31, 215, 221

Charity and health care 23–24, 27, 134

Church and social reform 112

Church and state 156–57

Church as community 107–10

Church/sect distinction 111–12

Churches and health care 153–72

Churchill, Larry 200

Churchill, Winston S. 50, 204

Civil law, role of 118–21, 154

Civil rights 123–26

Cleveland, William 43–44, 201, 203

Clifford, Clark 221

Clinton, Bill 195–98, 222

Cobb, John 215

Code orders 86–87, 92, 96

Common good 3, 97, 120, 122, 128, 129–33, 135, 144, 146–47, 187, 189–90, 215–16

Community 101, 103–22, 130, 134, 136

Commutative justice 134–35, 139

Confession 69

Conflicts of interest 35

Congregation for the Doctrine of the Faith 84, 164, 219

Connery, John 90, 209

Conscience clause 168

Constitution of U.S. 116

Consumer Choice Health Plan 40–42, 196, 203

Consumerism 63

Consumers' knowledge of health care needs 197

Contraception 35, 167–69

Cooperation in evil 153, 160–64, 218–19

Corporation 135

Cost of health care 17–23, 34, 82, 100, 130, 133, 175, 186, 189, 192, 211

Cost shifting 25–26, 200

Covenant loyalty 15–16, 107–09

Culture and health care 28–29

Cuomo, Mario M. 218

Curran, Charles E. 131, 138, 216, 219

Curzan, Nancy 210

DRGs 24–25, 53
DeLugo, Cardinal 82–83, 207–08
Dean, Howard 55
Death, meaning of 2, 11, 21–22, 61–64, 67–69, 99, 130, 142–43, 186–87, 189, 198, 200
Declaration of Independence 137
Declaration of Religious Liberty 126
Declaration of the Rights of Man 123
Declaration on Euthanasia 86–87, 94, 96, 199, 208, 210–11
Defense, national 118, 145, 175, 178–79, 182, 188
Defensive medicine 20–21, 127
Dialogue on national health care 189, 197–98
Dignity of persons 68, 85, 92, 94–95, 100, 110, 124, 126, 142, 145, 155, 166, 184, 186, 190–91
Dike against sin 154
Disinterested love 143
Distributive justice 3, 5–6, 11, 122, 128, 136–42, 173, 176, 191, 211
Dougherty, Charles 200
Drive-in clinics 34
Drug companies 193
Durable power of attorney 93

Ecology, environment 75–77, 127, 130, 187
Economic justice 112, 199, 216–17
Education 12, 30, 132, 144, 146, 174, 188, 217
Egalitarian justice 137–39
Embodiment 114
Emergency Rooms 27

Enthoven, Alain 41–42, 196, 203, 222
Entitlements 124, 127
Ethical and Religious Directives 168, 182, 206
Ethnicity and health care 4, 143–44, 180, 185
Eucharist 89
Euthanasia 63–64, 71–72, 91, 97–101, 171, 186, 211
Evans, Robert 177, 204

Faith and health care 103–05, 110, 113–115
Family 92–94
Fee for service system 19–20, 33, 54
Fein, Rashi 45, 203
Final Exit 63, 205
Finitude 61, 67, 75–77, 130, 144, 160, 188, 191
First Amendment 167
Formal cooperation 160–61
Free market 39, 49, 181
Friedman, Emily 199–201, 204
Futility 65, 95–97, 145, 147–48, 210

Gender and health care 12, 146, 165, 190, 221
Genetic research 171, 200
Geography and health care 12, 35–36
Ginzberg, Eli 201
Glendon, Mary Anne 127, 214
Global budgeting 53, 126
Globalization of health care 191–92
Goodness of society 116, 119, 132, 155, 174
Government, role of 116, 123–

25, 131, 136, 148–150, 177–79, 194

Grace 115–16

Gradual health care reform 1, 166, 174, 180

Grave inconvenience 82

Great Britain 50–51, 128, 149, 181, 200, 219

Green, Ronald 202

Gross National Product 29–30, 52–53, 196, 202

Gustafson, James 75–76, 207

Häring, Bernard 212

Harris, Louis 184, 201, 221

Hauerwas, Stanley 120

Hawaii 54

Health Access America 40, 203

Health Maintenance Organizations 16, 19, 33–34, 43, 48, 181, 183

Health Security Partnership 45, 203

Health USA Act 46, 203

Health care professionals 75, 98, 112, 121, 146, 153, 167–68

Health care reform 32, 79, 100–04, 106, 110, 112, 114, 120, 126, 129, 158, 164–198

Health care reform proposals 37–50, 150, 195–98

Hehir, J. Brian 206, 221

Heritage Foundation 38, 202

Heschel, Abraham J. 79, 207

Hilton, Bruce 201

Himmelstein, David 47, 200, 203

Hollenbach, David 216

Hospital and hospitality 65, 77, 109, 212

Howard, Coby 57

Human care setting 110

Human goodness 116

Human rights 3, 68–69, 114, 122–29, 174, 216

Humphry, Derek 205

Hunthausen, Raymond G. 219

Iacocca, Lee 30

Imagination 135, 174, 193–94, 222

Immigrants 35

Immortality of soul 61, 64, 68

Immunity from harm 124, 127–28

Immunizations 22, 187

Income of health professionals 18–19

Income tax on all 43–44, 48

Incompetent patient 93

Individualism 95, 103, 110, 126–127, 123–33

Infant mortality 11, 199, 221

Instrumental value of life 72

Jackson Hole Group 196, 220

Jesus Christ and healing 106–07

Job 66

John XXIII, Pope 126, 129, 149

John Paul II, Pope 76, 125, 130–31, 149, 205, 207, 215, 221

Johnson, Magic 219

Joint ventures 35, 202

Just war 73, 135, 145, 159, 206

Justice in health care 54, 56–57, 61, 66, 69–70, 72, 74, 85, 92, 94–95, 99, 100–02, 114, 118, 120–21, 129, 133–147, 154–55, 174–76, 178–79, 185, 188, 190–92, 197

Kelly, Gerald 82–83, 207–209

Kennedy, Edward 40–41, 44, 203

Kern, Rosemary 199, 201, 203

Kerrey, Robert 46, 52, 176, 200, 203
Kierkegaard, Sören 198, 222
King, Martin Luther 114, 213
Kirkman-Liff, B.L. 200–01
Kronick, Richard 41–42, 203
Kübler-Ross, Elisabeth 205

Laborem Exercens 149, 215, 217
Langan, John 206
Legal justice 135–36, 139, 143
Leo XIII, Pope 125, 127
Liability insurance 20–21
Liberal arts 78
Liberal theory of rights 123–24
Life as sacred 69–74
Limits to health care 141–42, 144, 146, 188, 221
Linton, Adam 53, 204
Lippmann, Walter 132
Lister, Joseph 128
Living wage 125, 134, 136, 142
Living will 93
Locke, John 123, 129
Lomas, Jonothan 177, 204
Lonergan, Bernard 221
Long term care 41, 43–44, 53, 183
Long, Crawford 128
Lottin, Odon 213
Love of neighbor 113–114
Luker, Kristin 220
Lumen Gentium 108
Lundberg, George 1, 199
Luther, Martin and Lutheranism 118–19, 154–55, 176, 213, 217

Maguire, Daniel C. 216
Maida, Adam 216
Maine 55, 204
Malpractice 21, 196, 200

Managed competition 42, 44, 196–97, 222
Maritain, Jacques 130–215
Marxism 130, 142
Maryland Catholic Conference 84
Massachusetts 54–55
Mater et Magistra 149, 217
Material cooperation 35, 160–64, 168, 219
May, William E. 90, 209
McCann, Dennis 131, 215
McCormick, Richard A. 84, 90, 207–09, 211, 218
McIntyre, Alasdair 120
McKibben, Bill 207
McMillan, Elizabeth 202
Medicaid 13–14, 37–44, 46–48, 55–56, 94, 288, 295, 200
Medical utopianism 21–22
Medicare 10, 13–14, 24, 27, 37–44, 46–48, 94, 175, 182, 195, 200
Mediplan 43–44, 203
Meilander, Gilbert 90, 209
Meritarian justice 140, 142
Metz, Johannes B. 206
Minnesota 55, 204
Mixed economy 124
Monotheism 105, 211
Mooney, Christopher 218
Moral principles 94–95, 97–98, 101–02, 116, 126, 154–56, 159, 177
Murphy, Charles 214
Murphy, Thomas 211
Murray, John Courtney 3, 132, 218
Mystery 104, 106, 212

National Leadership Commission on Health Care 40, 42–43, 203

Natural law 77, 115–18, 131, 177
Neal, Maria Augusta 206
Nebraska 46–47
Need for care and justice 142–43
Netherlands 98
Networks for delivery of care 182–83, 196
New York 55
New world order 192
Newborns, critically ill 5, 23, 206, 207
Niebuhr, H. Richard 132, 211, 213, 217
Niebuhr, Reinhold 117, 132, 160, 177, 213, 218, 220, 221
Non-discrimination 146
Novak, Michael 217
Nuclear arms 67, 112, 117, 191
Nutrition/hydration 5, 83, 88–93, 206–07, 209–10

O'Connor, John 169–71, 218–20
O'Rourke, Kevin 219
Optional health insurance 146, 179–80, 197
Ordinary and extraordinary means 2–3, 13, 82–84, 98
Oregon 32, 56–57, 144, 188, 198, 204–05
Organ transplants 189
Original sin 68
Outka, Gene 140–43, 146, 216
Overtesting 20–21
Overtreatment 68, 94, 99–101, 186

Pacem in Terris 126, 129, 214–15
Pain management 82, 87, 92
Paris, John 90, 98, 207, 209, 211

Participation in society 126, 130, 133, 146, 189
Pastoral care 65
Patient Self-Determination Act 94
Patient dumping 25
Paul VI, Pope 125, 214
Pennsylvania bishops 90–91, 207, 209–10
People of God 108
Pepper Commission 44, 195, 203
Perfect societies 157
Persistent vegetative state 89–93, 207, 209–10
Physicians for a National Health Program 47–48, 51, 200, 203
Pius XI, Pope 125, 138, 148–49, 214
Pius XII, Pope 72, 118, 126, 158, 206, 212, 218
Play or pay 38, 41, 43, 54–55, 165–66, 178, 195
Pneumonia 88
Pope John XXIII Center 90
Populorum Progressio 149, 214
Poverty, income, and health care 12, 128, 141–42, 146, 170, 176, 185, 195, 197
Pratt, Loring 203
Prayer 65, 68, 77
Pre-existing health condition 15–16, 200
Preferential option for the poor 3, 138, 143, 145, 154, 165, 185
Preferred provider organizations 16, 34
Premarital abstinence 168–69, 219–20
Prenatal care 22–23, 41
Presumptions 89, 93

Preventive medicine 22, 47, 187
Private delivery of health care 181–183
Private health insurance, state of 14–15, 19–20, 176
Private property 125
Private reform initiatives 32–33, 118, 119, 131, 136, 148–50
Prohibition 156
Prolongation of life 72–74, 96, 144, 198, 206, 209
Proportionality 73, 84, 88, 92, 94–96, 98, 100, 186
Prospective payment 25, 44–45, 47
Proximate and remote cooperation 161
Proximate solutions 117, 160
Public high risk pools 16, 111
Public order 131, 154
Public sponsors 42, 196–97

Quadragesimo Anno 148–49, 214, 217
Quality assurance 34, 100
Quality of life 73–74, 130
Quinn, John R. 169, 218, 220

Race and health care 11, 144, 146, 158, 165, 176, 180, 185
Rahner, Karl 62, 66, 78, 105, 205–07, 212–13, 221
Ramsey, Paul 81, 97, 140–41, 205, 207, 210, 216
Rare diseases 191
Rationing of health care 26–27, 50, 53, 56–57, 142, 144–48, 188–92, 211, 216
Rauschenbusch, Walter 211
Rawls, John 140
Reagan, Ronald 24, 36, 202
Recombinant DNA 78

Religion and public policy 153–72
Religious communities and health care 109, 112
Repentance 69
Rerum Novarum 125, 214
Research and experimentation 22, 73, 75–77, 192–93
Resurrection of Jesus 69–71
Resurrection of the body 61
Reverence for sick 77
Ricoeur, Paul 194, 222
Right to health care 123, 127–29, 135–36, 184, 214–15
Rockefeller, John D., IV 44, 203
Rommen, Heinrich 213, 218
Roosevelt, Franklin D. 214
Russo, Marty 48–49, 51, 178, 204, 220
Ryan, John A. 3, 112, 136–37, 211

Sacraments 109–110, 119
Sanctity of life 73, 129
Saranac Lake 81, 207
Satisfaction with health care 1, 31, 51–52, 221
Scandal 162
Science 77–79
Sectarian Christians 111–12
Self-discipline 187
Sex education 168–69
Sexuality 63, 115, 117, 154, 164, 167–71
Sickness as human event 64–66, 142
Similar treatment and justice 142–43, 215
Simon, William E. 217
Sin 67–69, 116, 123, 154, 160, 177
Single payer system 45–50, 53,

55, 176–80, 188, 195, 197, 220

Small businesses and health care 16, 42, 49, 177

Smith, Adam 123

Social Accountability Budget 24

Social Justice 126, 138, 197

Social and economic rights 124–25, 128

Social reform 116, 119, 214

Social responsibility 103, 139

Socialism 125, 149

Socialization 122, 148–150, 178–79

Socialized medicine 49–51, 181

Sollicitudo Rei Socialis 76, 125, 149, 207, 214

Soto, Domingo 82, 207

Sovereignty 192–93

Soviet Union 192

Sparks, Richard 85, 206, 208

Specialization in medicine 18

St. Louis *Post-Dispatch* 49

Standard of care 128, 136, 142, 145, 176, 184–85, 191, 197

Stark, Fortney 43–44

Starr, Paul 202, 205

States and health care 45–46, 54–57, 180–181, 197

Sterilization 35, 161–164, 167–68, 219

Stewardship of health resources 94–95, 100, 176

Subsidiarity 122, 148–150, 179

Substituted consent 92

Suffering 66–67, 99

Suicide 63–64

Supreme Court 93, 159

Synod of Bishops 126, 214

Tax credits and health care 38–40

Tax deduction of health care cost 165–66

Tax on employers 41–43, 45–46, 48, 54–55

Tax on providers 55, 177

Taxes and health care 135–36, 139–40, 143, 177–78

Technical feasibility of law 157–60, 171

Technology and health care 17, 22, 65, 68, 75–76, 79, 84–85, 91–93, 95, 97, 99, 101, 133, 142–44, 158, 187, 190, 192

Test tube babies 26

Theological anthropology 61, 79, 103–04, 113

Theology and health reform 105

Thomas, Clarence 63, 116

Thoreau, Henry David 141

Triage 141

Trinity 104, 106, 211–12

Tripartite approach to health insurance 40–43

Troeltsch, Ernst 11–12, 213

Trudeau, Edward L. 81, 99, 207

Truman, Harry S. 13, 178–79

Tuberculosis 81

Two realm theory 118

UNAC Program 42

US Economy and health care 29–31, 170, 177–78

Ulshafer, Thomas R. 218

Uncompensated care 23–24

Underinsured 10–11, 99–100, 105, 173–74

Undertreatment 187

Unenforceable laws 157–58

Uninsured Americans 2, 10–12, 99–100, 105, 139, 165, 173–74

United Nations 192–93
United Way 163
Universal Declaration on Human
    Rights 129
Universal Health Act of 1991
    48–49, 51, 203
Utilitarian justice 141–42
Utilization review 34, 100

Vatican II 71, 103, 108, 126,
    131, 205, 212, 214
Veatch, Robert 205, 208
Vermont 32, 55, 204
Virtue 120–121, 128
Vitalism 84
Vittorio, Francisco 82, 207

Vocation of health professionals
    71
von Nell-Bruening, Oswald 148

Wainwright, Geoffrey 207
Washington, State of 63, 68, 175,
    209, 211
Waxman, Henry 40–41, 49, 203
Welfare mothers and children
    166, 219
Williams, Oliver 215–16
Wofford, Harris 37
Woolhandler, Steffie 47, 200, 203
World Council of Churches 129
World peace and health care 191

Youngner, Stuart 208